Certified Occupational Therapy Assistant COTA®

Official NBCOT® Study Guide

for the

COTA Certification Examination

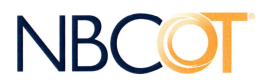

National Board for Certification in Occupational Therapy, Inc.
12 South Summit Avenue, Suite 100
Gaithersburg, MD 20877

www.nbcot.org

NBCOT ... your essential credentialing organization

Mission
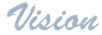

Serving the public interest by advancing client care and professional practice through evidence-based certification standards and the validation of knowledge essential for effective practice in occupational therapy.

Vision
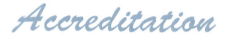

Certified occupational therapy professionals providing effective evidence-based services across all areas of practice worldwide.

Accreditation

NBCOT has been awarded organizational accreditation by the American National Standards Institute (ANSI) to the International Standard (ISO 178024) for organizations that offer Personnel Certification programs, NBCOT is also accredited by the National Commission for Certifying Agencies.

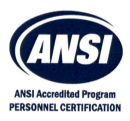

ANSI Accredited Program
PERSONNEL CERTIFICATION

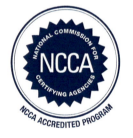

National Board for Certification in Occupational Therapy, Inc.
12 South Summit Avenue, Suite 100
Gaithersburg, MD 20877

http://www.nbcot.org

Printed in the United States of America.
ISBN 978-0-9910328-0-8

Foreword

The National Board for Certification in Occupational Therapy, Inc. NBCOT® is pleased to publish the newest edition of *The Official NBCOT Study Guide*. The occupational therapy content of this guide is aligned to the examination test specifications of the most current CERTIFIED OCCUPATIONAL THERAPY ASSISTANT® (COTA) Practice Analysis Study. This study identifies the domains, tasks, and knowledge required for occupational therapy practice.

The purpose of the COTA study guide is to:

- Provide a comprehensive overview of what you can expect during the examination.
- Include practice-focused sample items that mirror ones you may see on the actual examination.
- Outline strategies you can use when preparing for this high stakes examination.

We hope the information contained in this guide supports and augments your overall examination preparation activities. We know the practice of occupational therapy is constantly evolving. NBCOT uses only current information in examination items used for certification purposes. Although the information contained in this guide is current at the time of publication, you must be certain to refer to the most recent editions of references when studying for the NBCOT exam. While the information and practice items contained in this guide can assist your overall study efforts, it does not ensure or guarantee a passing score on the examination.

Best of luck as you pursue your professional career as a CERTIFIED OCCUPATIONAL THERAPY ASSISTANT!

Paul Grace, MS, CAE

President and Chief Executive Officer, NBCOT

Table of Contents

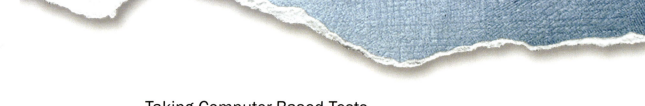

Introduction

Historically, regulation of the health professions in the United States began with a necessity to protect the public from the under-educated and under-trained professional. Over time, licensure, credentialing and certification have continued the tradition of protecting the public but have also increased their scope of activity to continuously improve the quality of practice in the profession.

Certification is a process by which key required competencies for practice are measured, and the professional is endorsed by a board of his/her peers (Barnhart, 1997). Earned certification means an individual has met a specified quality standard that reflects nationally-accepted practice principles and values (McClain, Richardson & Wyatt, 2004). The purpose of awarding the credential – CERTIFIED OCCUPATIONAL THERAPY ASSISTANT COTA® – is to identify for the public those persons who have demonstrated the knowledge and the skills necessary to provide occupational therapy assistant services. Certification has become the hallmark credential for professionals in a variety of industries, often serving as a benchmark for hiring and promotion (Microsoft, 2003). For more than 70 years, the COTA "mark" has been recognized by agencies, employers, payers, and consumers as viable symbols of quality educated and currently prepared practitioners.

NBCOT uses a formal process to grant the certification credential to an individual who: 1) meets academic and practice experience requirements; 2) successfully completes a comprehensive examination to assess knowledge and skills for practice; and 3) agrees to adhere to the *NBCOT Candidate/Certificant Code of Conduct*.

Overview and Purpose of the Study Guide

This study guide has six sections:
- Section 1 contains information about adult learning including critical thinking, learning as an adult, scheduling time for study, and controlling the study environment.

- Section 2 examines strategies for developing successful study habits such as using memory effectively, avoiding procrastination, and utilizing cooperative learning techniques.

- Section 3 considers general test-taking strategies including things to do before, during, and after the test, overcoming test anxiety, and guidelines for answering multiple-choice questions.

- Section 4 refers to exam specifics, including how NBCOT uses the results of practice analysis studies to guide test construction, format of the COTA examination, and overview of multiple-choice test items including how to deconstruct exam questions. The section also covers information on exam administration.

- Section 5 contains 100 multiple-choice COTA sample items representative of the domains and task areas found in the COTA test blueprint. Although the items included in the study guide practice test are grouped by domain areas to illustrate the type of questions that may be representative of a particular domain, questions on the actual certification examination will not appear grouped by domain, but will be randomized. *None of the questions included in this study guide will appear on the NBCOT certification examination.*

- Section 6 contains an answer key, the rationale for the correct response to each sample multiple-choice item, an explanation of why the remaining responses (distractors) in each item are incorrect, and a reference indicating where additional information about the item topic is located.

Appendix A includes the 2012 Validated Domain, Task, and Knowledge Statements for the CERTIFIED OCCUPATIONAL THERAPY ASSISTANT COTA certification examination. Appendix B includes a reference list of entry-level texts commonly used to reference COTA examination items. Appendix C provides a listing of standard abbreviations and acronyms used on the certification examination along with the associated expansion words. Appendix D includes a listing of common diagnoses/conditions, intervention applications/equipment, service delivery components and settings used on the certification examination.

This study guide is one of a number of official NBCOT study tools designed to assist candidates with their exam preparation. NBCOT does not guarantee enhanced performance on the NBCOT certification examinations for those using these products. However, the official NBCOT study tools are the only OTR and COTA certification examination study tools designed exclusively by NBCOT test development professionals and include sample practice questions written to the same psychometric standards as the actual NBCOT certification examinations.

> NBCOT does not administer, approve, endorse, or review preparatory courses relating to the NBCOT certification examinations or study materials produced by other vendors.

SECTION 1:
Adult Learning

Thinking Critically

Learning to think critically is one of the most significant activities of adult life (Brookfield, 1987). Indeed, it can be argued that without critical thinking, the individual views the world through a single, isolated lens, with no awareness of how others view their actions, or respect for the way others behave or make decisions about their world. To think critically is to become open to alternative ways of looking at, and behaving in, the world. As Brookfield (1987) reminds us, it is through critical thinking that we learn to pay attention to the context in which we (and others) think, act, and behave.

Critical thinking should be a core skill for all successful occupational therapy practitioners. It is through critical thinking that the occupational therapy practitioner creates and recreates aspects of the client's life. Critical thinkers are innovators, concerned with the potential for improvement while at the same time, respecting diversity of values, behaviors, and structures that guide the client's world. Critical thinking entails continual questioning of assumptions and an ongoing appreciation of the context in which life occurs. For example, the occupational therapy practitioner will appreciate that a person who has recently become a wheelchair user will experience an array of thoughts and emotions associated with this newly acquired mobility device. The person may feel happy that this device is enabling them to gain access into their community. On the other hand, they may feel embarrassed, or frustrated for others to see that they are having to rely on a mobility device to do the things that they were previously able to do.

All occupational therapy entry-level curricula seek to develop critical thinking skills to prepare their students for successful future practice. However, the skill of critical thinking can also be used as an important strategy for studying and preparing to take high stakes examinations such as the NBCOT COTA certification examination. The following provides a framework of how to apply critical thinking to your studying routines:

1. *Define what it is that you want to learn.* You may be familiar with the anatomical implications of ulnar nerve palsy for example, but want to know more about how this impacts thumb mobility and the challenges posed by this condition for a homemaker caring for a young child. In this sense, you could use critical thinking to help you appreciate the perspective of this homemaker. Define your learning into simple phrases such as:

   - How does the impairment affect the homemaker's ability to button the baby's clothes?
   - How might this impact ability to carry out grooming tasks?
   - Would adaptations be needed to open packets of formula?

2. *Think about what you already know about the subject.* Critical thinking will help you to identify strengths and gaps in your knowledge. Tapping into your previous experiences from fieldwork, labs, case studies, and readings, will give you a foundation upon which to build your learning. It will also help you to identify any prejudices that may be coloring the way you are currently conducting your studying. For example, you may be reluctant to invest much time in considering how you might design a pre-vocational skills program for someone with a substance abuse disorder if you have an underlying prejudice about people who abuse alcohol. Addressing these prejudices will enable you to view situations with an open mind, and aid your studying and ongoing journey towards successful future practice.

3. *Identify resources*. Critical thinking is about recognizing and using all the resources available to you. In this sense, consider resources in the widest possible context, have an open mind. These are a few you may consider, expand on these and design your own list:

- People – professors, fieldwork educators, mentors, peer group, community members
- Materials – textbooks, journal readings, reflective journals, class notes, lab exercises, videos, DVDs or Internet-based search engines
- Environments – fieldwork, community facilities, specialist clinics, adaptive workplaces, inpatient services

4. *Ask questions*. Use your critical thinking skills to enhance your understanding. Do you hold underlying beliefs about this disorder and is this influencing your studying? Does this author have prejudices about the information they are presenting? Is this professor telling you the full story about what it is like living with this disability? Continue to ask questions – why/what/how/if...

5. *Organize the information you have gathered*. Use your critical thinking skills to examine patterns and make connections across your learning. For example, you have reviewed your understanding about ulnar nerve palsy, talked to an occupational therapy practitioner who has provided services to people who have this condition, discussed ways this condition may affect household occupations with your peers, and identified possible short-term and long-term treatment goals from key texts.

6. *Demonstrate your knowledge*. Pulling all this information together, think of ways to demonstrate what you now know. Use lists, flowcharts, and summary statements to highlight key information. Discuss comparisons and similarities of disorders and strategies for overcoming occupational challenges. Write up an assessment report with recommendations for therapy.

Learning as an Adult

Through your occupational therapy education, you will have identified that there are many different ways to learn information. You will also be familiar with evaluating and selecting the most appropriate learning strategy to meet the needs of the clients you are working with. You can use the same strategies to help you identify the best ways for you to learn information in order to help you study for the certification examination.

As an adult learner who has engaged in a comprehensive program of study to prepare for a career in occupational therapy, you will recognize that these are some of the ways you have most likely approached your learning:

- Taken a self-directed approach
- Drawn upon a reservoir of life experiences that serve as a resource for your studying
- Driven by a need to know, do, or find out something new
- Utilized problem-centered, or creative problem-solving strategies to trigger learning experiences
- Been intrinsically motivated to learn as a way to reaching your goal to become an occupational therapy practitioner

It is not unusual however, particularly during transition stages (like preparing to take the certification examination!), for learners to question and re-evaluate their motivation for learning. If you take an adult learning approach to these questions and re-evaluations, it will help you to tap into previous strategies for effective learning, and assist you with renewing your motivation for study.

The following is a list of helpful strategies that reflect adult learning principles:

- *Plan your study.* Take an active role in planning your studying by setting realistic study goals and expected time commitments.
- *Evaluate your progress.* Check off your study goals regularly, demonstrate your knowledge, continually question, and reward yourself for a job well done.
- *Be open to new experiences – people, resources, materials, and environments.* Think outside of the box, who or what could help you learn more about what it is like to have this disability?
- *Recognize the value of past experiences.* Recall experiences from your fieldwork, group discussions, and creative projects. Make connections between these and new learning opportunities.
- *Develop an awareness of what helps you learn best.* Exploit these methods. For example, you may recognize that being able to discuss information in a group helps you to assimilate information. From this, you organize a weekly study group that focuses on preparing to take the certification examination.
- *Don't be afraid to ask for help.* Academic counseling centers, learning centers, writing centers, reading and/or study skills centers, and student service centers, are just a few resources available to students studying in professional academic programs. Adult learning embraces the notion that it is appropriate to ask for guidance to assist with the learning experience.

Scheduling Time for Studying

A common student complaint is that there is not enough time to go around. The time pressures involved in being an adult learner pursuing an occupational therapy education is enormous. Not only does the student typically face tightly scheduled classes, he or she is also expected to carry out several hours of preparation for each hour spent in the classroom, along with studying for tests and writing assignments. This, along with fieldwork and other community-based learning activities, soon add up to a full-time occupation. Many students in an entry-level occupational therapy program find that they have additional commitments related to employment and family/social responsibilities taking up even more of their time each week.

The way a student uses time, or wastes time, is largely a matter of habit patterns. By the time a student is ready to graduate from an occupational therapy program and start preparing to study for the certification examination, these study habits should be well-developed. Inefficient study habits can be changed however, and it is worth reviewing strategies for time scheduling here, reinforcing adult learning principles of taking responsibility for managing time when studying for the certification examination.

Use the following strategies to help schedule your time for studying:

- *Plan enough time for study.* Review the way you have planned your time to prepare for key assignments during your occupational therapy education. Think of occasions when you achieved a particularly successful grade or outcome, assess the factors that contributed to this including the amount of time you dedicated for preparation. In terms of the preparation you covered, knowledge that was being tested, and type of test/assignment given, estimate in hours/days how much preparation you carried out for this test. Now compare this to the certification examination. What are the similarities and differences between the two tests/assignments? Begin to formulate how much time you will need to optimally study for the certification examination. You are your own best estimator, you know how you work, and how much time you will need to prepare and plan for a successful study schedule. Be honest and realistic with your estimation.

- *Study at the same time each day.* To develop effective study habits, or modify inefficient study routines, it is recommended that students schedule certain hours that are used for studying throughout the day, every day. This enables a habitual, systematic study routine to develop and helps to maintain an active approach to learning and preparing for the test.

- *Make use of free time.* There are many opportunities throughout the day when you could take advantage of additional study time. Carry around a small notebook with the lists, summary statements, and flowcharts you have developed from your studying of specific occupational therapy practice. Use time between classes, riding the bus, waiting for appointments, walking on the treadmill to review your notes. Tap into your critical thinking, question your notes, jot down alternative explanations.

- *Schedule relaxation time.* Just as your occupational therapy training has emphasized the need for occupational balance, you should build in relaxation time into your study schedule. It is more efficient to study hard for a definite period of time, and then stop for a few minutes, than attempt to study on indefinitely. Plan for a 10-15 minute break after every 60-90 minutes of focused study. During this break time, ensure that you move away from your study materials, stretch, and use your other senses such as listening to music or drinking a glass of water, to give your mind a rest from the focused studying. Be disciplined however, to return to your study materials after each allocated break period.

- *Review regularly.* On a weekly basis, review the progress you have made towards reaching your study goals. Are you still on schedule? Do you need to build in additional study time? Is there flexibility in your schedule to allow for unforeseen events? This review time should prompt you to acknowledge just how well you are doing and build your confidence in preparing to take the certification examination.

- *Build in time for longer periods of occupational balance.* As well as taking short breaks between periods of focused study, plan for longer periods of "away time" when you can engage in enjoyable activities. Use these scheduled activities as a reward for reaching your study goals and as a way of nurturing your body before returning to your set study schedule.

Controlling the Study Environment

As an adult learner, you not only need to take responsibility for scheduling time for studying, you need to take control of your study environment. Your occupational therapy education has emphasized the importance of considering the environment in which your clients perform their daily occupations. You can apply the same skill to meet your own needs when designing a study environment to enhance your preparations for taking the certification examination. The following is a list of such environmental strategies:

- *Set aside a fixed place for study.* This ensures that over time, this place becomes associated with studying behavior, and it will be easier for you to engage in study activities.

- *Identify factors that increase your ability to focus.* For some people this means making the room as quiet as possible, for others this means putting on some background music. Check if the room is a comfortable temperature, that you have sufficient drinks/snacks close at hand, that your phone is turned off, and that you have all the materials you will need for studying.

- *Be goal-oriented.* Post the goal or goals associated for your planned study session next to your work desk. This will help you to focus and be an effective motivational tool.

- *Get in the study frame of mind.* Use symbols, or rituals, to get you in the studying frame of mind. This might include wearing a particular article of clothing or jewelry, reading a motivational quotation, looking at a favorite picture, or organizing your workspace. Whatever the action, the symbol/ritual will over time, become associated with studying behavior.

- *Refocus when needed.* If your mind starts to wander, stand up and look away from your study materials. Reconnect with the symbol/ritual you used at the start of your study session. Return refreshed and ready to refocus.

- *Build in regular review periods.* Post times above your desk when you plan to stop and verbalize what it is you have been studying.

- *Put other thoughts aside.* Keep a reminder pad beside you while you study. Use the pad to jot down thoughts if your mind begins to wander onto other activities besides your studying. Once you have written down the thought, return to your studying. This action will help you to refocus, while at the same time, provide a reminder to you later of things you have to do.

SECTION 2:
Study Habits

Section 1 of this guide considered adult learning and encouraged the reader to use adult learning principles, such as critical thinking, as a way to organize and conduct studying for the certification examination. This, along with specific emphasis on taking responsibility for managing time and the study environment, provides a strong foundation on which to develop effective study habits. This next section gives an overview of specific study habits. While it is not intended to be an exhaustive list you are encouraged to use the list as a trigger for examining your current study habits, and as a springboard for considering alternative study methods.

Effective Habits for Studying

(Adapted from Covey, S. R. (1989). The 7 Habits of Highly Effective People. New York: Simon & Schuster.)

- *Take responsibility for yourself.* Tapping into the principles outlined in the section on adult learning, remind yourself that in order to succeed, you need to make decisions about your priorities.

  Ask yourself questions such as:
  > *What interventions do I need to study this week?*
  > *How much time should I spend reviewing my knowledge on spinal cord levels?*
  > *Would it be helpful to coordinate my notes on major mood disorders with the case notes I gathered from my mental health fieldwork?*

- *Center yourself around your needs.* Remind yourself, "What is important to me now?" The certification examination can be viewed as the ending of one journey, and the gateway to your next journey. That is the end of your academic journey and the start of your professional occupational therapy career. It should be a natural step in your progression towards your chosen career. Use these thoughts to motivate as you set up your study schedule.

- *Follow up on priorities.* Keep to your schedule as far as possible. If you have fallen behind, take steps to review your progress and highlight the reasons for falling behind. For example, did you set unrealistic study goals or allow others to interrupt your studying? Try and build in methods to overcome these difficulties in the future, such as:
  > *Reviewing exam preparation goals*
  > *Revising your study schedule to ensure the goals are manageable*
  > *Ensuring the times you set-aside can be undisturbed*
  > *Informing others ahead of time about your undisturbed study time*

- *Congratulate yourself regularly.* Remind yourself of the progress you have made to date – the classes, fieldwork, labs, assignments, and tests completed up to this point. Use your study schedule and completed study goals to highlight the progress you are making towards your goal of taking the certification examination.

- *Consider other solutions.* If you are having difficulty understanding readings from textbooks and class notes, think of alternative ways for you to make sense of this material. For example, you might consider talking it through with one of your professors, revisiting a fieldwork site, or joining a peer study group.

Concentrating When Studying

Just as we all have the ability to concentrate, there will be times when it is difficult to remain focused. Our mind may wander from one topic to another, worries about the consequences of not doing well on the test, allowing outside distractions to interfere with study routines, and finding the material difficult or uninteresting can contribute to loss of concentration while trying to study. There are two effective methods for increasing ability to concentrate.

1. *Scheduled Worry Time.* Set aside a specific time each day to think about the things that keep entering your mind and interfere with your studying. When you become aware of a distracting thought, remind yourself that you have a specific time to think about them. Let the thought go, and keep your appointment to worry or think about those distracting issues at the time you have scheduled for these. Let your mind return to focus on your immediate activity of studying.

2. *Be Here Now.* When you notice your thoughts wandering, say to yourself, "Be here now." Gently bring your attention back to where you want it to be – your notes on developmental milestones, for example. If your mind wanders again, repeat the phrase "Be here now." and gently bring your attention back. Continually practice this technique and you should notice that the period of time between your straying thoughts gets a little longer each time. Be patient and keep at it.

Using Memory Effectively

While acronyms (invented combination of letters), acrostics (invented poems or sentences where the first letter of each word is a cue to an idea you need to remember), rhyme-keys, and chaining are recognized techniques for recalling systems or lists of information (and they are described at length in many other generic study guide texts), they are perhaps not the most effective methods for studying and recalling material in preparation for the NBCOT certification examination. Test items on this examination rely on candidates demonstrating their knowledge as it applies to the practice of occupational therapy.

Alternative methods should include using memory of situations and experiences as applied to practice.

For example, when studying the ulnar nerve, the student may associate actions of the flexor muscles with specific tasks such as holding a pencil or utensil. Fieldwork experiences may also act as a strong memory aid where students recall working with a particular individual who had a similar disability to the ones presented on the examination.

Using memory in this sense will enable you to apply your knowledge to the practice of occupational therapy.

Thinking Aloud

Through your learning about human development during your occupational therapy education, you are probably familiar with the term "private speech." Private speech is an accepted way for infants and children to think aloud or say what they are thinking as a way of demonstrating knowledge. Children use private speech to practice words, express ideas, form sentences, and as a way to make sense of their external world. Thinking aloud is essential to early learning. As we grow older, thinking aloud or private speech, becomes internalized. However, whenever we encounter unfamiliar or demanding activities in our adult lives, we can use private speech as a way to overcome obstacles and acquire new skills.

The more we engage our brain on multiple levels, the more we are able to make connections and retain what we learn. We can apply these same techniques to our study habits. As well as reading, we can create images, listen, talk with others, and talk with ourselves about the concepts we are learning. Some of us like to talk things through with someone else as a way of increasing our understanding, and others do not need another person around to talk with in this process. Using multiple senses and experiences to process and reinforce our learning is an individualized process, but one that can be very effective in helping to understand and retain knowledge.

Avoiding Procrastination

Procrastination can stop you from achieving the study goals you wish to reach. Here are some ways to help overcome procrastination:

Ask yourself, "What is it that I want to do?"

- What is your final objective, the end result?

    I want to review my notes on occupational therapy frames of reference.

- What are the major steps to get there?

    I need to locate my class notes.

    I need to check out the theory book from the library.

    I need to access my fieldwork journal where I wrote a case study using three major frames of reference.

    I need to prepare a grid showing the major frames of reference for my study group.

- What have you done so far?

    I've got the book from the library.

    I've found my fieldwork journal.

    I've bought some large sheets of grid paper and marker pens.

Next ask yourself, "Why do I want to do this?"

- What is your biggest motivation?

    I want to have all the frames of reference clear in my mind.

    I'd like to apply theoretical concepts to practice application.

    I need to feel I am contributing to the study group.

    I want to feel prepared for the certification exam.

- What other positive results will flow from achieving this goal?

    I can talk about my knowledge during recruitment interviews.

    I can use them to aid in selecting appropriate intervention activities in the future.

    I can assist members in my study group to understand the similarities and differences between the theories.

List what stands in your way:

- What is in your power to change?

    If I choose to review a frame of reference that I'm interested in first, it will help me to feel motivated to study the others.

    I don't want to prepare this grid in case I mess it up, but if I draft it on the computer I can build it up gradually.

    There are so many to cover, I'll never get through them all. If I group them together into categories, they will be more manageable for me to study.

- What resources beside yourself do you need?

    I could use some help with drawing up this grid.

    I am going to ask one other member from the study group to work on this with me.

    I am going to look on the NBCOT website to identify study tools available.

- What will happen if I don't progress?

    I won't know this material.

    There will be questions on the examination that I can't answer.

    I will let my study group down.

- Develop your plan:

    Set realistic goals for yourself.

    Define how much time each goal will take to realize.

    Reward your progress.

    Build in time for review.

    Visualize yourself succeeding!

- Admit to mistakes:

    Everyone makes mistakes. It is part of the learning experience.

    Distractions happen. Build extra time into your study schedule, and try to refocus on the task.

    Acknowledge frustration. We all get frustrated at times, especially when things are not going as well as we had planned. Turn that frustration around, and acknowledge that you are doing something about it.

Index Study Systems

Using index study systems is an effective strategy to evaluate how well you know and understand the material you have studied. Follow these steps to build up your own index study system:

- As you read through your study notes, write down potential test questions about the material on one side of an index card.

    How does macular degeneration affect a person's ability to complete grooming tasks?

    What recommendations could the occupational therapy practitioner make to a homemaker with macular degeneration?

    What type of assistive devices would be beneficial for a person with macular degeneration?

- On the other side of the card, write an explanation to answer your questions. Include references or texts from your academic studies to validate your response.

    A person with macular degeneration will have difficulty distinguishing visual details such as variations in color, patterns and contrast. Activities such as medication management, putting on make-up, or selecting clothing may be difficult for the person to complete.

    (Reference: Early MB. (2013). Physical Dysfunction Practice Skills for the Occupational Therapy Assistant. (3rd ed.). St Louis, MO: Elsevier Mosby. Pages 440-441).

- When you have completed writing up a series of index cards about a particular subject, shuffle the cards. Look at the card on top and read the question. Try to answer it in your own words. If you experience difficulty, turn the card over and review the answer you have written.

- Keep going through the deck until you know all the information you have catalogued.

- Carry the cards with you – take advantage of free time to review your knowledge.

- Use the cards to study with your peer group. Test each other, check that others understand your explanations, come up with alternative solutions to the problems posted.

Cooperative and Collaborative Learning

Your occupational therapy education has provided many opportunities for you to experience cooperative and collaborative learning opportunities. This is an interactive learning approach where group members develop and share a common goal, contribute understanding of specific problems, post questions, offer insights and solutions. Many students find it effective to use a similar approach for studying to take the certification examination.

What makes an effective study group?

- Use understanding of group process principles.

- Keep the group to a manageable size (maximum of six).

- Assign a group leader.

- Choose members who will bring specific strengths to the group.

- Empower members to contribute.

- Encourage commitment.

- Share group operating principles and responsibilities such as:

  ○ Commitment to attend, preparation, and starting meetings on time.

  ○ Having discussions and disagreements that focus on issues, not personal criticism.

  ○ Taking responsibility to share tasks and carry them out on time.

Process of setting up a study group:

- Set goals, define how often and with what means you will communicate, evaluate progress, make decisions, and resolve conflict.

- Define resources, especially someone who can provide direction, supervision, counsel, and even arbitrate.

- Schedule review of your progress and communication to discuss what is working, and what is not working.

SECTION 3:
Test-Taking Strategies

The previous section presented an array of strategies to encourage effective study habits. This section examines general test-taking strategies including what to do before, during, and after the test, tips for overcoming test anxiety, and guidelines for answering multiple-choice items.

Before, During, and After the Test

Before the test:

Remind yourself of the progress you have made to date. You have already completed an occupational therapy program. You have taken many academic courses, successfully completed assignments, and passed several major tests. Think back to how much you knew about occupational therapy at the start of your program, compared to how much you know now. View the certification examination as just one step further towards your goal of becoming an occupational therapy practitioner. You have taken many steps up to this point, and this is one of the last steps you will need to take towards your career goal.

Continue to set realistic study goals. Identify your strengths and address any weaknesses in your knowledge. Regularly review your progress, check off your study goals, seek additional help for information you are finding difficult to understand, build in regular breaks, and try to predict how the information you are studying might be presented on the test. Remember that items on the certification examination are mostly practice-based. Although knowing lists and memorizing facts are helpful, you must be able to apply that information to a practice-based situation. Use your study notes, index card systems, study groups, lists, charts, and review papers to learn how to apply this knowledge to practice across a variety of settings and with a variety of conditions.

The night before the test:

- Do not engage in last minute cramming. If you have followed a well-planned study schedule, there is no need for you to do last minute cramming.
- Make sure you know the exact site of the examination center. Estimate how long it will take you to get there and build in extra time for traffic, taking the wrong turn, unforeseen circumstances. Make sure your vehicle has gas, and is in full working order.
- Make sure you have all the documentation you will need to take with you to the test site – refer to the latest copy of the NBCOT Candidate Handbook online at www.nbcot.org.
- Engage in some form of physical activity. This will help to alleviate pretest nerves.
- Decide what clothes you plan to wear – comfort and layered clothing are key considerations.
- Try to get a good night's sleep, and remember to set the alarm clock.

The day of the test:

- Arrive at the test site early.
- Try not to talk to others taking the same test – anxiety can be contagious.
- Take some deep, slow breaths.
- Remind yourself how well you have done up to this point.

- Organize your workspace – familiarize yourself with the computer and ensure you can see the clock on the screen.

- Ask for headphones if you know you will be distracted by others working around you.

- Ask the proctor for a marker board to use during your test time.

- Ensure your seat feels comfortable, and sit in an upright position.

- Advise the test proctor of any problems or concerns you have regarding the test environment prior to beginning the test.

During the test:

- Take the tutorial. Time for taking the tutorial is NOT deducted from your actual exam time.

- Divide up the time you have been given for the test. The COTA exam consists of 200 multiple-choice items. Divide the time you have for the exam (4 hours unless you have been granted special accommodations) by 200. Build in time so you can review the entire test prior to finishing. Make a note of your progress at the end of every hour so you can keep yourself on schedule.

- Use the marker board provided to help you organize and clarify your thinking.

- Change your position regularly – stretch, drop your shoulders, open and close your fingers, shift in your chair.

- Read the instructions VERY CAREFULLY before starting to answer the multiple choice questions.

- When answering multiple-choice items:
    - Use the "Mark" button on the computer screen to review items later if time permits.
    - Only change an answer you have initially selected if you are really sure it is an incorrect response. The answer that comes to mind first is often correct.
    - Rely on your knowledge and do not watch for patterns. The test answers are randomized.

- Don't panic if other people in the room finish before you do. You do not need to leave the room until you have used all of the allotted time.

- If you experience a technical problem during the exam, inform the test center proctor.

After the test:

- Resist the urge to talk through test items and potential answers with your peer group. You have completed the exam, and it is too late to change your answers now.

- Resist the urge to open up your study notes, texts, and review guides for the same reason given above.

- Remember, it is against the NBCOT Candidate/Certificant Code of Conduct to discuss test items with other candidates, or to record test information from memory.

- Relax. You have waited for this moment for a long time, you can do no more, reward yourself for completing this stage.

- If you do wish to post an exam challenge, ensure you do this in writing, and within the timelines given in the NBCOT Exam Candidate Handbook.

Overcoming Test Anxiety

It is of course, very natural to experience a level of anxiety prior to sitting for the certification examination. This is a day that you have been working towards for a long period of time, and marks your passage towards achieving your career goal. Your occupational therapy education has provided you with many instances when anxiety has been a natural response—interviewing your first real patient, arriving at your first day of fieldwork, giving a formal presentation in front of a large audience. Remind yourself that a certain amount of anxiety can actually be very beneficial to your performance. It heightens your awareness and enables you to remain alert. Anxiety can become a problem however, if it lasts too long and starts to interfere with your ability to concentrate.

The following are some tips to help you manage your anxiety:

- Prepare, prepare, prepare. This includes following a realistic and well planned study schedule, as well as preparing physically for getting to the test site on time.
- Ensure you have exercised, eaten, and had a good night's sleep.
- Use cue cards to remind you how well you have done.
- View the test as an opportunity to demonstrate how much you know and have achieved.
- Remember, the examination is not designed to trick you.
- Engage in relaxation techniques – visualization, controlled breathing, tensing and relaxing muscles groups.
- Change position, visit the restroom, have a drink of water.

If you notice that at times you have not been able to manage your anxiety levels, and that this has interfered with your ability to perform on exams, seek help from a qualified professional. Your student counseling center, or healthcare provider will be able to recommend help available to you.

SECTION 4:

Specifics of the NBCOT COTA Examination

Background

Following certification industry standards NBCOT certification examinations are constructed based on the results of practice analysis studies. The ultimate goal of practice analysis studies are to ensure that there is a representative linkage of test content to practice, making certain the credentialing examination contains meaningful indicators of competence, and providing evidence that supports the examination's content validity of current occupational therapy practice. The periodic performance of practice analysis studies assists NBCOT with evaluating the validity of the test specifications that guide content distribution of the credentialing examinations. Because the practice of occupational therapy changes and evolves over time, practice analysis studies are conducted by NBCOT on a regular basis.

NBCOT conducted a practice analysis study of certified occupational therapy assistant practice in 2012. The results from this study were used to construct examination test blueprints for examination administrations starting in January 2014.

Building upon previous studies, a large-scale survey was used with entry-level COTA practitioners who were asked to evaluate job requirements on criticality and frequency rating scales. The job requirements were classified as the domains, tasks, and knowledge required for current occupational therapy assistant practice.

- Domains broadly define the major performance components of the profession.
- Tasks describe activities that are performed in each domain (i.e. things that practitioners do).
- Knowledge statements describe the information required to perform each task competently.

Table 4.1: Sample of a domain, task, and knowledge statement for the COTA:

Domain: Assist the OTR to acquire information regarding factors that influence occupational therapy performance throughout the occupational therapy process.
Task: Provide information regarding the influence of current condition(s) and context(s) on occupational performance in order to assist the OTR in planning interventions and monitoring progress throughout the occupational therapy process.
Knowledge: Activity analysis in relation to the occupational profile, practice setting, and stage of occupational therapy process.

The results of the survey were analyzed to identify the most critical and frequently performed tasks by the COTA survey respondents. Weights were then established to determine the relative proportion of test items devoted to each of the three domain areas established for the COTA examination blueprints. Appendix A displays the COTA Validated Domain, Task and Knowledge Statements derived from the results of the 2012 NBCOT practice analysis study. These statements comprise the test blueprint and will guide examination development for the NBCOT COTA certification examinations beginning January 2014.

The percentage of items in each domain area is shown in Table 4.2. These percentages remain constant on each exam form of the COTA certification examination. As mentioned above, there are multiple task and knowledge statements for each of the three over arching domain areas.

Table 4.2: COTA Blueprint Specifications Based on the 2012 Practice Analysis Study
(Effective for COTA Examinations Administered January 2014 Onward)

Domain	Domain Description	% of Test Items
01	Assist the OTR to acquire information regarding factors that influence occupational performance throughout the occupational therapy process.	32%
02	Implement interventions in accordance with the intervention plan and under the supervision of the OTR to support client participation in areas of occupation throughout the occupational therapy process.	60%
03	Uphold professional standards and responsibilities to promote quality in practice.	8%

Exam Construction

NBCOT examinations are "high stakes" examinations. To ensure the defensibility of these examinations, NBCOT applies multiple levels of quality controls during every aspect of the item and examination development process. Additionally, NBCOT contracts with a professional testing agency to ensure adherence to rigorous psychometric standards for the development, delivery, and scoring of the certification examinations.

Each item (question) appearing on the COTA examination has been developed to assess essential knowledge acceptable for entry-level performance by an occupational therapy assistant. In addition, the items are designed to differentiate from an individual whose knowledge is acceptable for certification and an individual whose knowledge is not acceptable for certification. All items have been subjected to multiple rigorous reviews. Examination items are carefully reviewed for bias, making sure that the context, setting, language, descriptions, terminology, and content of the items are free of stereotype and equally appropriate for all segments of the candidate population.

The NBCOT exams include a pre-selected number of field-test items on each test form. Although these items are not considered when scoring candidates' exams, performance data is collected and analyzed. This statistical analysis is an important quality control step that NBCOT uses to preserve the reliability of the examinations. Candidates are not able to distinguish between the scored and unscored items. Once a sufficient number of responses are collected on an item, the item statistics are reviewed based on pre-determined metrics. Items meeting these metrics are entered into the bank of items that can be used as scored items on subsequent exams. Item-level statistics falling below these metrics are used to flag items that need additional review and revision before undergoing further levels of field-testing.

In summary, scored items are only included on the examination if they: 1) satisfy the examination blueprint specifications resulting from the practice analysis study, 2) meet development standards described above, or 3) satisfy specific psychometric standards.

Format of the COTA Examination

The COTA examinations are comprised of 200 multiple-choice items based on blueprint specifications. Some of the items may contain a picture or chart. Candidates can take an optional tutorial about the functionality of the test screens at the start of the examination. The four-hour test clock starts at the conclusion of the tutorial.

Multiple-Choice Test Items

Each multiple-choice test item starts with a stem or premise. This is usually in the form of a written statement or a question. Stems always relate to tasks and knowledge required for entry-level COTA practice. The following is an example of a stem:

An OTR and a COTA with established service competence are collaborating to evaluate a kindergarten student who has autism. Which task can the COTA complete as part of this INITIAL data gathering process?

Following the stem, there are four possible response options. From the four options, there is only ONE correct response. The other three options are distractors. Distractors typically represent common fallacies or misconceptions about the item topic. In the sample provided, there is only one choice that represents the task the COTA with service competence is able to do within scope of practice guidelines. You need to solicit the best response based on all the information presented in the stem. The following are the four possible response options posted for the example above:

> A. *Score a sensory integration assessment.*
> B. *Select a developmental assessment to administer.*
> C. *Document evaluation outcomes of a classroom observation.*
> D. *Administer a standardized developmental checklist.*

In considering the response options provided, you should ask, "What is this question *really* asking?" The question above is testing the knowledge of scope of practice guidelines related to acquiring client information as part of a school-based evaluation. You must also recognize the student is in kindergarten and has autism and this is part of the INITIAL data gathering process in collaboration with the OTR. Response option "A" is incorrect because a sensory integration assessment can only be administered by an OTR specially trained to give the test. Option "B" and Option "C" are incorrect because these should be completed by the OTR as part of the initial assessment. Response option D is correct because it is within the scope of practice for a service competent COTA to administer a standardized checklist.

Although there is never more than one correct answer in a multiple-choice item, you may find it difficult to choose among the four plausible options. If this is the case, re-read the stem and identify the key words such as "MOST EFFECTIVE", "INITIAL", "FIRST", or "NEXT". Boldface words in an item stem provide information to help guide your decision-making about the correct answer. The following sample item illustrates this:

A patient in an acute care facility had an uncomplicated total hip replacement, anterolateral approach one week ago. What movement of the affected hip is typically **CONTRAINDICATED** *based on standard hip precautions?*

> *A. Abduction beyond 25°*
>
> *B. External rotation*
>
> *C. Flexion to 90°*
>
> *D. Internal rotation*

The correct response is option "B". Total hip precautions for an anterolateral approach include the following restrictions: hip external rotation, hip extension, hip adduction (crossing legs or feet). Options "A," "C" and "D" are movements that are safe to complete during this stage of rehabilitation.

Now let's dive a little deeper and look at a more systematic approach to answering multiple choice items. This process is called "deconstructing a multiple choice test question".

DECONSTRUCTING A MULTIPLE CHOICE TEST QUESTION

As mentioned in the previous section, the key to answering multiple choice questions, is being able to identify what the question is *really* asking. This is especially important when answering questions that test your critical reasoning skills – where there are several plausible options presented. If you are having difficulty identifying the one *BEST* correct answer and cannot make up your mind between two answer options, try the following steps to help deconstruct the question:

> Step 1: Carefully read the question stem.
>
> Step 2: Identify the topic of the question.
>
> Step 3: Start eliminating some of the answers.
>
> Step 4: Revisit Step 1 again.
>
> Step 5: Select the correct response.

Putting it into Practice!

Start by carefully reading the question stem:

A client sustained a distal radius fracture 8 weeks ago. The client has been participating in outpatient OT 3 times per week for the past 6 weeks and has been making steady progress toward goals. During the past two sessions, the client has reported a progressive increase in pain when completing functional tasks. What **INITIAL** action should the COTA take based on this information?

    A. Reduce the intensity of the intervention activities used during scheduled sessions.

    B. Ask the OTR to complete a reevaluation and update the intervention plan.

    C. Decrease the frequency of the intervention sessions until the pain subsides.

    D. Gather information from the client about symptoms and recent activity patterns.

STEP 2 Identify the topic of the question

    A. What is the practice setting?

    B. What are we told about the client (e.g., diagnosis, length of time in hospital, changes in status)?

    C. Based on the condition, what would we be expecting to see?

    D. What alarm bells are going off based on the information being presented in the stem?

    E. What are your immediate thoughts?

    F. Underline/highlight key information being presented in the stem.

    G. Which words are bolded indicating very important actions the COTA needs to take?

A client sustained a distal radius fracture 8 weeks ago. The client has been participating in outpatient OT 3 times per week for the past 6 weeks and has been making steady progress toward goals. During the past two sessions, the client has reported a progressive increase in pain when completing functional tasks. What **INITIAL** action should the COTA take based on this information?

Our review here indicates that the client sustained a distal radius fracture 6 weeks ago, and is participating in outpatient OT. The client has been making steady progress until the last two sessions. The alarm bell in this case is the length of time since fracture, and the report over the previous two sessions about increased pain during activities. Our immediate thoughts should be that it is not unusual for a client to have some pain or discomfort associated with the healing process. But, since this pain is progressively worsening, it is important to determine if the client reinjured the hand or has been overusing the hand during daily tasks. Therefore, the **INITIAL** action the COTA should take is to gather more information from the client about the symptoms and current activity patterns. Now that you have formulated some thoughts about what **INITIAL** action the COTA should take, look at each of the response options to start eliminating some of the answers.

STEP 3 Start eliminating some of the answers

Which response option can you strike off right away?

    A. Reduce the intensity of the intervention activities used during scheduled sessions.

    B. ~~Ask the OTR to complete a reevaluation and update the intervention plan.~~

    C. Decrease the frequency of the intervention sessions until the pain subsides.

    D. Gather information from the client about symptoms and recent activity patterns.

We can immediately strike off option "B". Although the COTA should collaborate with the OTR if indicated, the COTA should **INITIALLY** gather more information about the client's condition and activities prior to consulting with the OTR to recommend a complete reevaluation and to update the intervention plan.

Now that option "B" is eliminated, look at response option "A".

    A. Reduce the intensity of the intervention activities used during scheduled sessions.

    B. ~~Ask the OTR to complete a reevaluation and update the intervention plan.~~

    C. Decrease the frequency of the intervention sessions until the pain subsides.

    D. Gather information from the client about symptoms and recent activity patterns.

This option indicates the COTA should change the intervention activities. This may be an option if the pain is not typical for this phase of the healing process. But, the COTA does not have enough information about the client's condition or the cause of the pain to make this determination. This is therefore not the action that the COTA should take INITIALLY.

That leaves us to choose between options "C" and "D".

    A. ~~Reduce the intensity of the intervention activities used during scheduled sessions.~~

    B. ~~Ask the OTR to complete a reevaluation and update the intervention plan.~~

    C. Decrease the frequency of the intervention sessions until the pain subsides.

    D. Gather information from the client about symptoms and recent activity patterns.

STEP 4 Let's go back to the question stem and make sure we understand what this question is really asking.

The client is participating in outpatient OT after having a distal radius fracture 8 weeks ago.
The client has been making steady progress until the last two sessions.
The client reports progressive increase in pain during functional tasks.
What **INITIAL** action should the COTA based on this report?

A client sustained a distal radius fracture 8 weeks ago. The client has been participating in outpatient OT 3 times per week for the past 6 weeks and has been making steady progress toward goals. During the past two sessions, the client has reported a progressive increase in pain when completing functional tasks. What **INITIAL action** should the COTA take based on this information?

A. Reduce the intensity of the intervention activities used during scheduled sessions.

B. Ask the OTR to complete a reevaluation and update the intervention plan.

C. Decrease the frequency of the intervention sessions until the pain subsides.

D. Gather information from the client about symptoms and recent activity patterns.

0	1	2	3	4	5	6	7	8	9	10
	C	*A*		*B*					*D*	

Option "D" is the *BEST* answer. Based on evidence and the information presented in the item question, this option is the **INITIAL** action the COTA should take based on the client's report.

Options "A" and "B" should be done only if indicated after the COTA gathers more information from the client about the symptoms and recent activities.

Option "C" should only be done by the OTR if indicated after gathering more information from the client.

Using the scale with "0" representing an incorrect decision and "10" representing the BEST option, the "distractors" (response options A, B, C) cluster at the lower end of the scale. Response option "D" falls at the high end of the scale based on the evidence and considering all of the information presented in the question.

* References: Hussey S, Sabonis-Chafee B, Clifford O'Brien J. (2007). Introduction to Occupational Therapy (3rd ed). St. Louis, MO: Elsevier Mosby. Pages 178-179.

Early MB. (2009). *Mental Health Concepts and Techniques for the Occupational Therapy Assistant* (4th ed.). Baltimore, MD: Wolters Kluwer –Lippincott, Williams & Wilkins. Page 585.

Standard Setting, Equating, and Scoring

All NBCOT certification examinations are criterion referenced. This means in order to pass the examination, the candidate must obtain a score equal to – or higher than – the minimum passing score. The minimum passing score represents an absolute standard and does not depend on the performance of other candidates taking the same examination. The minimum passing score on the COTA certification examination is set by content experts using widely recognized standard setting methodologies.

NBCOT uses a scaled scoring procedure to determine a candidate's final score. The scaled score is not a "number correct" or "percent correct" score. Raw scores are converted to scale scores that represent equivalent levels of achievement regardless of test form. The passing point for the COTA certification examination is set at 450 points with the lowest possible score set at 300 and the highest possible score set at 600 points. Candidates must obtain a scaled score of at least 450 points in order to pass the examination. Additional information about the psychometric principles NBCOT uses for certification examination development and scoring is located in the NBCOT publication titled: *Foundations of the NBCOT Certification Examinations*. This document can be viewed/downloaded from the "Publications" section of the NBCOT website (www.nbcot.org).

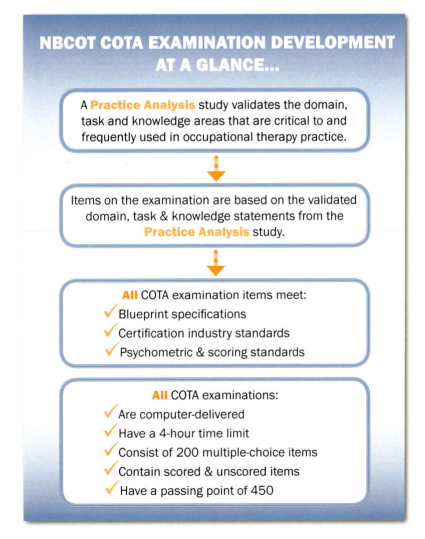

NBCOT COTA EXAMINATION DEVELOPMENT AT A GLANCE...

A **Practice Analysis** study validates the domain, task and knowledge areas that are critical to and frequently used in occupational therapy practice.

⬇

Items on the examination are based on the validated domain, task & knowledge statements from the **Practice Analysis** study.

⬇

All COTA examination items meet:
✓ Blueprint specifications
✓ Certification industry standards
✓ Psychometric & scoring standards

All COTA examinations:
✓ Are computer-delivered
✓ Have a 4-hour time limit
✓ Consist of 200 multiple-choice items
✓ Contain scored & unscored items
✓ Have a passing point of 450

Examination Preparation Tools

In addition to this study guide, NBCOT offers a variety of test resources to assist COTA candidates in preparation for the certification examination. Each tool reflects the validated domain, task and knowledge statements of the current examination blueprint. Additionally, these tools are the *only* COTA certification examination study tools designed exclusively by NBCOT test development professionals. Candidates can be confident these tools provide an authentic introduction to the types of questions appearing on the actual certification examination. For information related to the official NBCOT study tools, click on the "Study Tools Central" link on the NBCOT website home page (www.nbcot.org).

The NBCOT official study resources for the COTA candidate include:

- Entry-level Self-assessments
    - General Practice
    - Mental Health
    - Pediatrics
    - Physical Disabilities

- Content Tests
    - Mental Health
    - Pediatrics
    - Physical Disabilities

- Practice Tests
- Multiple choice sample items posted on NBCOT Facebook page

Taking Computer-Based Tests

Test centers are built to standard specifications. NBCOT candidates arriving at the test site must have appropriate documentation in order to be permitted to test. Candidates should check their Authorization to Test (ATT) letter for details of this documentation.

In addition to requiring proper documentation at the test site, NBCOT uses biometric-enabled check-in services at all test sites. This procedure consists of a number of steps to verify your eligibility to test, including taking an electronic record of your ID, photo imaging, and a digital fingertip record. You are required to undergo fingertip analysis any time you leave and re-enter the testing room for validation purposes.

Private modular workstations provide ample workspace, comfortable seating, and lighting (Figure 1). Proctors monitor the testing process through an observation window and from within the testing room. Parabolic mirrors mounted on the walls assist proctors in observing the testing process (Figure 2). All testing sessions are videotaped and audio-monitored. During the testing session, people taking examinations other than the NBCOT examinations may be in the testing room.

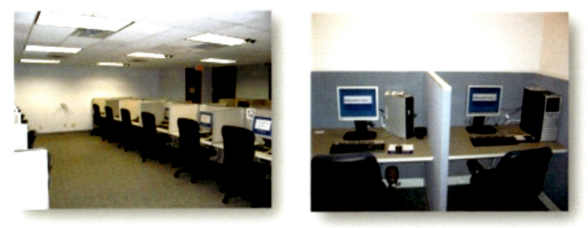

Figure 1: Prometric Testing Center Modular Workstations

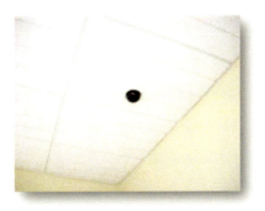

Figure 2: Parabolic surveillance mirrors inside Prometric Testing Centers

As mentioned in a previous section of this guide, the COTA examination consists of 200 multiple-choice test items. There is a tutorial at the beginning of the examination explaining the process of selecting responses to the examination items. Time spent on the tutorial does NOT count against the time allotted for the examination. Candidates are strongly encouraged to take the tutorial prior to starting the examination. Candidates are allotted four (4) hours to complete the entire examination.

A standard 14-point font is used for the screen text. When answering the multiple-choice items, you can use the "Mark" and "Unmark" buttons to flag items, and the "Review" button to return to marked items if time permits. If you run out of time, marked items that have responses will be counted for scoring purposes.

All test situations are subject to some noise and distraction. In a computer-based setting, other test-takers may be taking essay exams, so there may be some keyboarding sounds from test-takers nearby. Proctors are required to walk through the testing area periodically and test center staff may also be providing some brief assistance to other test-takers in the room. If a candidate is concerned that these situations may be distracting, the proctor can provide "noise-cancellation" headsets for the candidate to use while taking the exam.

Candidates may take a break, go to the restroom, or get some water or a snack from a locker. Breaks may be taken at any time, and as often as is reasonable and necessary. It is important to note that the exam time continues to run during any of these breaks. For more details on test administration, refer to the current copy of the NBCOT Certification Examination Handbook.

Accommodations

In compliance with the Americans with Disabilities Act (ADA), NBCOT makes special testing arrangements for candidates with professionally diagnosed and documented disabilities. Under the ADA, a disability is defined as "a physical or mental impairment that substantially limits one or more major life activities" (e.g., caring for one's self, performing manual tasks, walking, seeing, breathing, learning, working). If you intend to apply for special testing accommodations in order to take the COTA certification examination, you need to provide comprehensive documentation supporting your diagnosis, and the impact of the disability on major life activity. Submit the documentation AFTER you have filed your examination application. A review is then conducted per ADA guidelines. An Authorization to Test (ATT) letter will be sent only after the decision about the special accommodations request is final. Please refer to information about Special Accommodations online at www.nbcot.org.

Score Reports

Passing Candidates will receive by mail a congratulatory letter that includes the total scaled score on the examination, an official NBCOT® certificate and wallet card, and the *Credentials Essentials™ Toolkit*.

Failing candidates will receive an official score report that includes the total scaled score, along with performance information for each domain area of the examination. The information on the domain areas is provided for diagnostic purposes only. The score report will include information about how to register to retake the examination.

NBCOT only provides program directors with a list of the names of candidates who pass the certification examinations. In the event that an education program director requests a certification examination score, the exam candidate MUST grant permission to release his/her score. Candidates may do so by contacting NBCOT to request a *Candidate Score Report Release Form*.

See the NBCOT Certification Examination Handbook at www.nbcot.org for more details about score reporting.

Unfortunate Events

Examination Content Challenges, Administration Complaints, and Appeals

A candidate may submit an examination challenge, administrative complaint or an appeal of the examination score. Details on how to submit a challenge, complaint or appeal are outlined in the NBCOT Examination Candidate Handbook at www.nbcot.org.

Failing the Examination

Unfortunately, not every candidate who takes NBCOT's certification examinations will achieve a successful passing score. While it is obviously very disappointing for any candidate to receive notification indicating failure to meet the passing requirement (a scaled score of 450 points or above on the overall examination), it is essential to address the consequences of this occurrence. A candidate's test score (including a fail score) will only be reported to the candidate, and to a state licensing board, if the candidate requested for their score transfer reports to be sent to a state regulatory board(s). **Without the candidate's written permission, no other persons will be informed of the candidate's failed score.** Not passing the NBCOT certification examination may impact the candidate's plans to begin an occupational therapy assistant job position. If a candidate does not successfully pass the NBCOT certification examination and is negotiating with an employer about a COTA position, the candidate must inform the potential employer about the need to retake the certification exam. Additionally, candidates should contact state regulatory entities for specific information regarding temporary licenses.

Candidates who fail the certification examination will be informed when they are able to submit another exam application. After the exam application has been approved a new Authorization to Test (ATT) letter will be sent to the candidate specifying dates of the candidate's examination eligibility period.

Preparing to Retake the Certification Examination

There may be many reasons for a candidate failing the NBCOT certification examination. Reflecting on potential reasons is an important first step in preparing to retake the examination. These reasons may include:

- Poor test-taking strategies
- Inadequate study habits
- Lack of preparation
- Test anxiety
- External stresses

After identifying potential reasons, revisit the initial sections in this study guide to help develop a plan of action. Pay particular attention to the sections on Adult Learning, Study Habits, and Test-Taking Strategies. Use the domain-level information from your score report to reassess your knowledge. Review the information about "deconstructing" multiple-choice items. Use this method to supplement further review of the sample multiple-choice items and clinical simulation problems in this study guide. Familiarize yourself with the domain, task, and knowledge statements of the examination blueprint and focus further study on areas of weakness – considering a variety of practice settings and diagnoses.

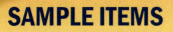

SECTION 5:

Sample Items

COTA Multiple-Choice Sample Items

The 2012 COTA Validated Domain, Task, and Knowledge Statements (see Appendix A) provide the basis for the COTA certification examination item development. The outline for the examination is based upon the three domain areas identified in the blueprint, and the percentage for each domain weight (the approximate percent of items from the domain appearing on each examination) is listed in Table 4.2.

This section consists of 100 COTA multiple-choice sample items across all three domain areas. Examples of domain-specific test items are grouped together under each domain heading for learning purposes in this study guide. However, candidates should take note that the items on the actual certification examination will appear in random order.

The following multiple-choice items are samples related to Domain Area 1:

> **Assist the OTR to acquire information regarding the factors that influence occupational performance throughout the occupational therapy process.**

1. Which symptoms typically have the **MOST** impact on self-feeding for a client who has stage 1 Parkinson's disease?

    A. Dysphagia and oral motor weakness

    B. Incoordination and bradykinesia

    C. Diminished protective sensation and strength

    D. Hypertonicity and spasticity

2. An inpatient with major depression was admitted to an acute psychiatric facility one day ago. A screening indicates the patient lives alone at home and recently retired after having worked as clergy in a church for the past 35 years. What information would be **MOST BENEFICIAL** to gather for contributing to the patient's occupational profile?

    A. Explore potential part-time vocational or volunteer opportunities in the area.

    B. Determine the patient's willingness to participate in a retirement support group.

    C. Ask the patient about options for contributing to church-sponsored activities.

    D. Use open-ended questions related to the patient's feelings about retirement.

3. A young adult client has mild cognitive impairment, poor attention span, and limited frustration tolerance secondary to a TBI. One of the client's goals is to resume work in a restaurant. The COTA is gathering information to contribute to the client's initial work readiness evaluation. Which data gathering method would be **BEST** for the COTA to use for this purpose?

    A. Administer a standardized vocational interest inventory.

    B. Interview the employer about the client's previous work habits.

    C. Assess cognitive-perceptual skills using simulated job tasks.

    D. Determine the client's physical capacity for work.

4. A client who has schizophrenia recently transitioned from living at home with parents to residing in a group home. The client is having difficulty adjusting to this new living arrangement. The COTA is interviewing the client and client's parents as part of the intervention planning process. What is the **PRIMARY** purpose for conducting this interview?

    A. To learn about the client's emotional needs

    B. To determine the client's developmental stage

    C. To become aware of the client's unconscious conflicts

    D. To identify the client's typical performance patterns

5. A client who has multiple sclerosis works as an administrative assistant in a large corporation. Fatigue and weakness interfere with the client's ability to complete job tasks. The corporate physician is requesting a job site analysis for this client. What is the **PRIMARY** purpose of this type of analysis?

    A. To observe the client interacting with co-workers within the office environment

    B. To determine the critical work demands in relation to client needs

    C. To assess the client's vocational interests in relation to work assignments

    D. To identify the management's willingness to provide special accommodations

6. What is the **PRIMARY** purpose for administering a standardized occupational performance survey to clients who are participating in an inpatient hand rehabilitation group activity?

    A. To determine clients' level of function through direct observation of BADL tasks

    B. To obtain subjective information about clients' vocational competency

    C. To track normative information about the impact of the injury on clients' life satisfaction

    D. To collect reliable information about clients' engagement in essential activities

7. A COTA is scheduled to lead a series of assertiveness training sessions for clients participating in a community-based mental health program. At the start of the first session, the COTA plans to administer a questionnaire asking the clients about situations in which they believe they are not assertive and want to change. What is the **PRIMARY** purpose for administering this questionnaire?

    A. To identify areas of strengths and weaknesses

    B. To promote socialization among group participants

    C. To determine issues the group participants want to address

    D. To evaluate the clients' self-assessment skills

8. A client has sensory-perceptual deficits secondary to a mild CVA. Motor skills remain intact. Which task would be **BEST** to ask the patient to complete when screening for tactile agnosia?

    A. Picking up objects from a tabletop

    B. Turning a water faucet on and off

    C. Distinguishing a key from a coin in a pocket

    D. Holding an eating utensil in the dominant hand

9. A COTA is administering a standardized test to assess perceptual skills of a client who had a recent CVA. After reading the instructions to the client, the client has difficulty initiating the task as requested. What action should the COTA take in response to this observation?

    A. Provide the patient hand-over-hand assistance to begin the task.

    B. Continue the test as indicated in the protocol manual.

    C. Ask the client to repeat back the protocol instructions.

    D. Repeat the test protocol instructions while demonstrating the task.

10. An inpatient has left hemiplegia secondary to a CVA 3 days ago. One of the patient's goals is to be able to bathe independently. What would be the **FIRST** step for supporting progress toward this goal?

    A. Review one-handed bathing techniques with the patient.

    B. Determine the patient's routines and current self-care abilities.

    C. Obtain detailed information about the patient's home set-up.

    D. Determine the patient's ability to use adaptive equipment.

11. A COTA is working with the Individualized Education Program (IEP) team to determine a student's eligibility for school-based OT intervention. Which information does the team rely upon for making final eligibility determinations?

    A. Physician's referral and diagnosis severity

    B. Standardized test scores and documented disability

    C. Classroom performance and curriculum-based needs

    D. Birth history and previous early intervention services

12. An older adult patient who had a recent CVA was admitted to an inpatient rehabilitation facility 2 days ago. The patient is scheduled to participate in an initial self-care session. A records review indicates the patient immigrated to the United States several years ago and is living with family members. What **INITIAL** action should the COTA take to support the patient's participation in the intervention sessions?

    A. Apply broad generalizations about the patient's culture to self-care activities.

    B. Gather information about the patient's cultural values regarding self-care.

    C. Ensure a translator is available for each of the patient's scheduled sessions.

    D. Administer a standardized evaluation to determine the patient's current function.

13. A client is participating in an activity group in a community-based mental health center. The group plans to make decorations for an upcoming traditional religious holiday event. The client refuses to participate in the task citing a conflict with personal religious beliefs. How should the COTA respond to the client's refusal?

    A. Encourage the client to respect the values of the other group participants.

    B. Suggest the client discuss reasons for refusing with a pastoral counselor.

    C. Explore specific reasons for the conflict between the activity and religious beliefs.

    D. Offer an alternate activity that is pertinent to the established goals.

14. A COTA is selecting activities to include in a homemaking skills session with a client who has an anxiety disorder. A review of the occupational profile indicates the client immigrated to the United States with a spouse and two children one year ago. Stress of the relocation and symptoms of the anxiety disorder are interfering with the ability to complete simple daily tasks. One of the client's goals is to fully participate in family roles and routines. What activities should the COTA include in the session in order to support the client's goal?

    A. Incorporate the client's culture and values into the session activities.

    B. Encourage the client to adapt to social norms of the United States.

    C. Provide instruction about using appliances typically found in homes in the U.S.

    D. Teach the client about the family values system in the United States.

15. A client who has schizophrenia is participating in a day treatment program at a community-based mental health center. During an OT group, the client admits to "forgetting" to take prescribed medications. After discussing the importance of taking the prescription medication with the client, What action should the COTA take **NEXT** in response to this comment?

    A. Contact the referring physician and report the client's noncompliance.

    B. Alert the client's family or significant other to monitor compliance.

    C. Teach the client to use a smart phone application for medication management.

    D. Have the client sign a behavioral contract agreeing to take the medication.

16. An inpatient is participating in a rehabilitation program after experiencing an exacerbation of relapsing-remitting multiple sclerosis. The patient is making steady progress toward the intervention goal of resuming independence with homemaking tasks. While completing personal laundry tasks during a session, the patient reports being extremely tired from not sleeping well the previous night and asks to take a brief rest. What action should the COTA take **INITIALLY** in response to the patient's report?

    A. Ensure the patient uses energy conservation techniques for the remainder of the session.

    B. Allow the patient to take a short break and encourage pursed-lip breathing.

    C. Discontinue the session and notify the charge nurse about the patient's fatigue.

    D. Demonstrate additional work simplification techniques to use during laundry tasks.

17. A client had a partial hand amputation secondary to an industrial accident 3 months ago. The client has been attending OT at least 3 times weekly since the date of injury. Until recently, the client has been very compliant with the home exercise program. Now the client is cancelling appointments and seems less motivated to complete prescribed daily exercises and splinting. Which action should the COTA take **INITIALLY** in response to the client's behaviors?

    A. Contact the client's case manager about the change in attitude.

    B. Discuss these observations and concerns with the client.

    C. Decrease the frequency and intensity of the overall intervention program.

    D. Review the treatment plan and long term goals with the OTR.

18. During an ADL group session, an inpatient with quadriplegia reports a sudden onset of a pounding headache, begins to perspire excessively, and has chills. What **INITIAL** action should the COTA take in response to these symptoms?

    A. Activate the facility medical alert system.

    B. Transport the patient to their room to rest.

    C. Stop the activity until the patient's vital signs stabilize.

    D. Recline the back of the patient's wheelchair.

19. A resident of a long term care facility has moderately severe cognitive decline secondary to dementia. The resident occasionally becomes combative during morning BADL. What **INITIAL** action should the COTA take when these behaviors occur?

    A. Allow for nursing staff to complete the dressing session.

    B. Identify the possible factors that provoked the behavior.

    C. Use a firm voice to tell the resident to stop the behavior.

    D. Delay the session until later in the afternoon.

20. A COTA is fabricating a splint for a client who recently had a deep partial thickness burn to the dorsum of the hand. When the COTA removes the bulky dressing, the patient becomes light-headed and begins to sweat. What **INITIAL** action should the COTA take in response to this occurrence?

    A. Break open an ammonia ampule and slowly pass it under the client's nose.

    B. Assist the client to a supine position and elevate the client's legs.

    C. Ask the client to rest their head on the table or between their knees.

    D. Moisten a cloth with cool water and hold it across the client's forehead.

21. Which of the following homemaking activities uses the **GREATEST** range of bilateral shoulder flexion and elbow extension?

    A. Ironing shirts and placing them on a hanger

    B. Washing dishes in a sink and drying pots and pans

    C. Folding sheets and hanging towels on a clothesline

    D. Dusting tabletops and vacuuming carpets

22. One of the goals of a client in a home health setting is to increase active shoulder flexion. As part of the intervention, the client removes collectible items from eye-level wall-mounted shelves, dusts the items and the shelves, and returns the collectibles to the shelves. What is the purpose for including this task as part of the client's intervention session?

    A. To simulate a variety of movement patterns

    B. To facilitate isometric muscle contractions

    C. To promote cleanliness within the home

    D. To use purposeful activity for promoting goals

23. The dining room aides of an assisted living facility has been receiving increasingly more requests to assist residents during mealtimes. The nurses report this is due to recent admissions of several residents who have low vision, and ask the COTA for recommendations for increasing residents' independence with feeding. What action would be **MOST BENEFICIAL** for the COTA to take based on this request?

    A. Complete a meal time observation to identify the residents' mealtime barriers and needs.

    B. Train the dining aides on how to respond to the residents' requests for assistance during meal times.

    C. Advise dining aides to serve food on brightly colored trays with each food group on a separate plate.

    D. Arrange dining room seating so at least one resident who does not have a visual deficit sits at each dining table.

24. An inpatient has hemiplegia secondary to a recent TBI and is functioning at Level V (Confused-inappropriate, Non-agitated) on the Rancho Los Amigos scale. A COTA is planning an initial dressing session to teach the patient lower body dressing techniques. Which intervention environment would be **MOST CONDUCIVE** for supporting the patient's success during this session?

    A. Quiet room in the rehabilitation department away from other patients

    B. Clinic gym so the patient can sit on a firm mat table for support

    C. Bathroom in the patient's room so the patient can sit on the tub bench

    D. Patient's private room with the patient seated in a bedside chair

25. An inpatient in a rehabilitation facility is in the recovery phase of Guillain-Barré syndrome. The patient is the parent of a 4-month-old infant. One of the patient's long term goals is to be able to lift the infant in and out of the crib prior to discharge in 3 weeks. The patient has met the initial goal of being able to lift a 10-pound (4.5 kg) weight from the floor to a table. Which statement represents an achievable short term goal to include as part of the intervention plan documentation for the **NEXT** phase of the patient's rehabilitation?

    A. "Patient will be able to use proper body mechanics to safely lift 15 pounds (6.8 kg) from the floor to the table 5 out of 5 times without assistance."

    B. "Patient will verbalize methods for using proper body mechanics for lifting objects over 50 pounds (22.7 kg)."

    C. "Patient will lift the infant from the floor to the patient's lap from a seated position in a standard wheelchair."

    D. "Patient will increase strength of both upper extremities by at least 2 pounds in one week."

26. A COTA working in a community-based mental health program has been working with a client who has a substance abuse disorder. Based on observation of the client's performance and a review of the client's goals, the COTA concludes the client has attained maximum benefits from attending a vocational skills group. Which action should the COTA take based on this information?

    A. Advise the client that OT is no longer indicated.

    B. Discuss the client's status with the supervising OTR.

    C. Re-evaluate the client prior to the next group session.

    D. Discharge the client from this particular group.

27. An inpatient has neurobehavioral deficits secondary to a CVA one month ago. At the time of the initial evaluation, the patient required moderate verbal cues to complete oral hygiene and grooming. Currently, the patient is able to complete these tasks independently during self-care sessions. This is one week earlier than the timeframe listed in the intervention plan for achieving this goal. What action should the COTA take prior to the **NEXT** scheduled BADL session with this patient?

    A. Revise the intervention plan with new short term goals.

    B. Administer a standardized functional assessment.

    C. Advise the physician of the patient's progress.

    D. Collaborate with the OTR to review the intervention goals.

28. A student in the fifth grade of school has moderate developmental delay and participates in school-based OT. The COTA is gathering information to provide to the OTR for the student's upcoming reevaluation. Which information is **MOST IMPORTANT** to obtain for this purpose?

    A. Cognitive abilities and verbal skills for vocational potential

    B. Motor performance compared to typically developing children of the same age

    C. Performance patterns during routine classroom activities

    D. Just-right challenges supporting the student's success in leisure activities

29. A multidisciplinary team in a long term care facility is developing a plan of care for a resident who has mild cognitive decline secondary to dementia. One of the objectives of the plan is to use a conservative approach for helping the resident manage urinary incontinence. What would be the **PRIMARY** role of the COTA in this process?

     A. To identify the impact of the incontinence on the resident's social interactions

     B. To recommend environmental and clothing adaptations for the resident

     C. To outline methods nursing can use to track the resident's bladder habits

     D. To teach the resident a program of biofeedback and pelvic floor exercises

30. A COTA working in an elementary school setting attends students' annual Individualized Education Program (IEP) planning meetings. What information would be within the scope of practice for the COTA to report during these meetings?

     A. Age-appropriate leisure activities the student should be able to complete

     B. Progress the student has made in school-related activities over the past year

     C. Results of recently administered standardized perceptual-motor tests

     D. Receptive and expressive communication skills the student currently uses

31. A COTA working in an outpatient setting is preparing a home program for a client who has mild hemiplegia and neurobehavioral deficits secondary to a CVA several months ago. What information would be **MOST IMPORTANT** for the COTA to verify prior to teaching the client the program?

     A. Extent to which the client has a detailed understanding of the program rationale

     B. Client's learning needs for independent follow through of the prescribed program

     C. Client's capacity to verbalize the home program instructions

     D. Amount of family support available to the client on a daily basis

32. An inpatient who has moderately severe cognitive decline secondary to Alzheimer's disease has been undergoing medical treatment for pneumonia. Currently, the patient has difficulty sequencing steps for self-care activities and becomes easily frustrated. The patient will be discharged in one week to live at home with adult children. What action should the COTA include as part of the overall intervention in preparation for the patient's transition to home?

     A. Advise the family to hire a home health aide to assist the patient with daily BADL tasks.

     B. Provide the family with behavioral strategies for supporting the patient's function at home.

     C. Recommend the family purchase assistive devices for the patient to use during BADL tasks at home.

     D. Instruct the family to adjust medication routines to prevent agitation and support the patient's function.

33. A patient was admitted to a rehabilitation facility due to a recent decline in function secondary to amyotrophic lateral sclerosis. One of the patient's goals is to live at home as long as possible. The COTA is gathering information about the patient to contribute to the initial discharge planning meeting. Which information would be **MOST IMPORTANT** to gather for this purpose?

    A. Patient's vocational and leisure history

    B. Current ROM and strength measurements

    C. Assisted living option for the patient to consider

    D. Durable medical equipment needs for ADL

34. An inpatient who has congestive heart failure has had a recent decline in function and now requires a wheelchair for mobility. A COTA is completing a home visit in preparation for the patient's discharge to live with family. The family live in an apartment on the second level of a multi-level apartment building. During the home visit, the COTA identifies several areas in the apartment that are not accessible by a wheelchair. What action should the COTA take **NEXT** based on this information?

    A. Collaborate with the patient and family to discuss the needs.

    B. Suggest ways furniture should be rearranged for wheelchair access.

    C. Have family members notify the apartment manager of needed changes.

    D. Assess the patient's ability to ambulate short distances using a walker.

35. An outpatient client, whose primary insurance is Medicare, sustained a wrist fracture 8 weeks ago and has been participating in OT 3 times per week for the past 2 weeks. ROM and strength of the affected extremity are improving and the client has returned to limited work in a department store. However, the client is still reluctant to use the hand. At the end of a session, the client refuses to schedule more OT visits citing "transportation problems". What action should the COTA take **INITIALLY** in this situation?

    A. Talk with the client to determine a solution.

    B. Teach the client an independent home program.

    C. Refer the client to a home health agency.

    D. Encourage scheduling a monthly reevaluation.

36. A COTA working in a long term care facility is responsible for teaching residents strategies for supporting their independence with BADL. During BADL sessions over the past week, several of the residents reported that the assistive devices used during the sessions are not available to them when completing routine BADL with the nursing aides. What action would be **MOST BENEFICIAL** for the COTA to take in response to these reports?

    A. Submit a incident report about the nursing aides to the appropriate supervisor.

    B. Advise the residents to ask for the assistive devices prior to starting BADL.

    C. Present in-service training to nursing staff about the benefits and uses of BADL devices.

    D. Ensure the assistive devices are in a visible location and labeled with the residents' name.

37. A COTA is preparing an in-service about injury prevention for employees at a data-entry and computer software company. Which information is **MOST IMPORTANT** to include as part of this presentation?

    A. Symptoms associated with cumulative trauma

    B. Isokinetic exercises for reducing painful symptoms

    C. Impact of work-related injuries on the company

    D. Methods for reducing work-related risk factors

38. The multidisciplinary team at a community-based program is developing a substance abuse relapse program. The focus of the program is to promote healthy alternatives for at-risk clients. What is the **PRIMARY** contribution of the COTA during the initial phase of program development?

    A. To recommend program topics unrelated to triggers that lead to misuse

    B. To identify resources for determining barriers to participation

    C. To suggest program activities related to leisure skill development

    D. To determine specific outcome measures for the program

39. A COTA is preparing to give a presentation for an arthritis support group. The goal of the presentation is to communicate the role of occupational therapy in assisting individuals who have systemic lupus. Which communication method would be **MOST BENEFICIAL** to use in the presentation in order to meet this goal?

    A. Describe specific OT assessments typically used with individuals who have lupus.

    B. Discuss OT interventions and service options for individuals who have lupus.

    C. Simulate a typical OT session by including one of the participants as an example.

    D. Demonstrate a range of exercises for individuals who have lupus.

The following multiple-choice items are samples related to Domain Area 2:

> **Implement interventions in accordance with the intervention plan and under the supervision of the OTR to support client participation in areas of occupation throughout the occupational therapy process.**

40. A COTA is selecting an activity for a group of children who are 3 years old and have mild developmental delay. The primary purpose of the group is to promote coordinated movements of both upper extremities. Which activity would be **MOST BENEFICIAL** for supporting the group goal?

    A. Rolling a large therapy ball to each other

    B. Playing dress-up to imitate action heroes

    C. Playing prone-lying scooter board games

    D. Jumping rope in rhythm to a well-known song

41. A 9-year-old child who has moderate hemiplegia often neglects to use the affected upper extremity. Which activity would be **MOST BENEFICIAL** for encouraging the child's bilateral fine motor control?

    A. Playing with a hand-held video game

    B. Tossing a beanbag at a target

    C. Playing a game of darts

    D. Drawing on a chalkboard

42. A student in the second grade has illegible handwriting. The student has good proximal control but poor fine motor control and uses a palmar grasp whenever holding a pencil. One of the intervention goals is for the student to learn to use a more mature pencil grasp when writing. Which activity would be **MOST BENEFICIAL** to include in the intervention for promoting progress toward this goal?

    A. Searching for small objects in a bucket of uncooked rice

    B. Finger-painting on a large pad placed on an upright easel

    C. Rolling out firm modeling dough on a table top

    D. Threading string through pegs on a vertically positioned pegboard

43. A student in the first grade has a mild visual perceptual deficit. The teacher reports the student is a good auditory learner but often writes letters and numbers backwards when completing class assignments. Which activity would be **MOST BENEFICIAL** for improving the student's directionality for writing?

    A. Playing a game of follow-the-leader to form letters in the air

    B. Having the student repetitively practice forming letters on paper

    C. Teaching the student to use rhymes that describe how to form letters

    D. Providing the student with worksheets to trace letters of the alphabet

44. A school-age child has severe tactile defensiveness secondary to congenital cortical blindness. The student will be participating in OT to improve sensory processing prior to learning Braille. Which activity should be included as part of the child's **INITIAL** intervention for supporting this objective?

    A. Object identification games with vision occluded

    B. Fun activities that reinforce pre-reading concepts

    C. Drills for assigning meaning to raised dots on paper

    D. Graded play using a variety of textured materials

45. A kindergarten student who has visual perceptual deficits is able to name letters of the alphabet, but has difficulty with the motor planning skills for writing the letters on paper. One of the intervention goals is for the student to improve writing legibility. Which activity would be **MOST BENEFICIAL** for the student to complete as a preparatory activity during the initial stages of intervention?

    A. Manipulate brightly colored magnetic letters on a vertical surface.

    B. Use firm resistance putty to shape letters of the student's first name.

    C. Place alphabet stickers in between the lines on a piece of paper.

    D. Copy letters from a template onto wide-ruled paper using a scented marker.

46. A 5-year-old child has moderate hypertonicity secondary to cerebral palsy. Increased muscle tone interferes with the child's ability to complete dressing independently. Which technique would be **MOST EFFECTIVE** for reducing the child's muscle tone prior to initiating a dressing task?

    A. Bouncing the child up and down on a large therapy ball

    B. Having the child gently rock forward and backward in quadruped

    C. Using quick tapping to the spastic muscle bellies

    D. Applying heavy joint compression to both arms

47. A 4-year-old child has hypotonia secondary to cerebral palsy. This results in poor lip closure which makes it difficult for the child to transition from using a bottle to drinking from a cup with a spouted lid. Which intervention would be **MOST BENEFICIAL** for the child to do in order to promote initial progress toward drinking from a cup?

    A. Sip a favorite fruit juice from a cup with a nose cut out.

    B. Blow soap bubbles into the air at the start of the session.

    C. Whistle a simple tune before each drink from a cup.

    D. Suck on a piece of sour candy prior to practicing drinking from the cup.

48. A student in kindergarten has moderate extensor tone secondary to athetoid cerebral palsy. The COTA is teaching the classroom aide how to move the student from the wheelchair to the floor so the student can participate in floor-time activities with other students. Which method is **MOST EFFECTIVE** for the caregiver to use for inhibiting the student's extensor patterns during this transfer?

    A. Support the student's trunk with one arm and abduct the lower extremity with the other arm.

    B. Hold the student facing forward with hips and knees flexed and neck slightly flexed.

    C. Have the student's back face the caregiver with hips and knees extended and neck slightly flexed.

    D. Position the student so the legs straddle the caregiver's hip.

49. A student in the fourth grade has mild developmental delay secondary to Down syndrome. The student has difficulty with tabletop writing tasks due to poor proximal stability. Which recommendation represents a compensatory strategy for enhancing proximal stability when writing?

    A. Allow the student to write in a prone position bearing weight on the forearms.

    B. Put a medium-sized triangular grip on the student's writing utensil.

    C. Have the student stand at a counter-height tabletop during writing tasks.

    D. Fasten a one-pound (0.45 kg) weight on the student's wrist during the writing task.

50. A 4-year-old child has persistent asymmetrical tonic neck reflex (ATNR) and symmetrical tonic neck reflex (STNR) secondary to moderate cerebral palsy. The COTA is teaching the caregiver strategies to use when feeding the child. The COTA positions the child in a chair that provides good head and trunk control. Where should the caregiver sit to inhibit the ATNR and STNR reflexes when feeding the child?

    A. Slightly on the right side of midline and just above the child's eye level

    B. Next to the child and at the child's eye level

    C. In front of the child and slightly below the child's eye level

    D. At the child's midline and slightly above the child's eye level

51. An adolescent sustained a C_8 spinal cord injury several months ago. One of the outpatient intervention goals is for the adolescent to be independent in functional mobility on all indoor surfaces and level outdoor terrain. What type of mobility equipment would be **MOST BENEFICIAL** for supporting this goal?

    A. Lightweight folding wheelchair with modified rims

    B. Power wheelchair with reclining back and chin control

    C. Adjustable wheeled stander with sip and puff switch

    D. Standard wheelchair with removable arms and leg rests

52. A kindergarten-age student who has spastic cerebral palsy is painting while seated at a table in art class. The student can hold a paintbrush, but a dominant asymmetrical tonic neck reflex prevents the student from reaching for the paint located near the student's dominant side. Which technique would be **MOST EFFECTIVE** to use for inhibiting this reflex in support of the student's success with the art task?

    A. Place the paint at midline in front of the student.

    B. Provide the student with a paintbrush with a weighted handle.

    C. Adapt the tabletop to a 45° elevated angle.

    D. Have the student use a standing frame while painting.

53. A client has recently been diagnosed with rheumatoid arthritis. The client works as a medical laboratory technician. Completing essential job tasks of frequently turning off equipment knobs and tightening specimen cup lids result in bilateral hand and wrist pain by the end of the work day. Which movements are **CONTRAINDICATED** for this client to use during these job tasks?

    A. Wrist extension

    B. MCP joint ulnar deviation

    C. Wrist ulnar deviation

    D. Composite finger extension

54. A client who had a CVA several months ago is baking cookies during an OT session. The client uses the correct amount of dough for each cookie, but places the dough only on the right side of the cookie sheet before stating the pan is ready to place in the oven. Which sensory processing deficit could be attributed to this behavior?

    A. Figure-ground neglect

    B. Homonymous hemianopsia

    C. Diminished depth perception

    D. Right-left disorientation

55. A COTA is selecting a craft activity for an inpatient who has cancer and has decreased platelet levels due to chemotherapy medications. Which craft material is **CONTRAINDICATED** for this patient to use?

    A. Burlap fabric or yarn

    B. Water-based paints

    C. Scented drawing markers

    D. Scrap booking cutting blade

56. A client has mild hemiparesis secondary to having a left CVA several months ago. One of the client's goals is to increase strength and fine motor control to be able to play the piano; a favorite leisure activity. Which activity would be **MOST BENEFICIAL** to include in the intervention for supporting progress toward this goal?

    A. Making a pinch pot using firm modeling clay

    B. Manipulating various size pegs and stringing one-inch (2.54 cm) beads

    C. Practicing a repetitive program of piano keyboard drills

    D. Completing resistive exercises while listening to piano music

57. Which of the following is **MOST IMPORTANT** for the COTA to do in preparation for a self-care session with an inpatient who has COPD?

    A. Arrange ADL supplies so they are within easy reach for the patient.

    B. Make sure the patient has adequate standing tolerance to complete the entire activity.

    C. Have the patient's preferred spray deodorants and talcum powders available for use.

    D. Place a chair just outside of the bathroom door in case the patient becomes fatigued.

58. A client who has reduced visual acuity reports difficulty preparing meals due to the low vision. Which kitchen modification would be **MOST BENEFICIAL** to include as a recommendation for supporting the client's participation with meal preparation tasks?

    A. Label food items in large print using high-contrast colors.

    B. Use fluorescent bulbs in household light fixtures.

    C. Keep frequently used items on the counter top.

    D. Replace wooden cabinet doors with glass panels.

59. A client has difficulty completing home management tasks due to symptoms associated with COPD. One of the intervention goals is for the client to learn techniques for reducing the impact of the disease symptoms on occupational performance. Which intervention should be included in the **INITIAL** phase of rehabilitation for supporting this goal?

    A. Teach the client to use energy conservation techniques during BADL tasks.

    B. Provide the client with a home program of upper body strengthening exercises.

    C. Have the client attend a series of stress management classes.

    D. Instruct the client how to use visual imagery techniques for pain reduction.

60. Which technique would be **MOST EFFECTIVE** for a client to use for managing the symptoms of COPD during a functional task at home?

    A. Breathing out when pushing items and breathing in when pulling items

    B. Inhaling through the mouth and exhaling through the nose when lifting

    C. Taking shallow quick breaths whenever shortness of breath occurs

    D. Crossing both arms across the chest when breathing becomes difficult

61. A client had surgery to decompress the ulnar nerve 2 weeks ago. The surgical incision is healing as indicated in the picture below. Which intervention should be included as part of the patient's scar management intervention at this phase of healing?

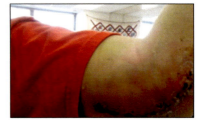

    A. Circumferential moist heat packs

    B. Continuous wave low intensity ultrasound

    C. Vibration using a high intensity mini-vibrator

    D. Lotion application and compression wrap

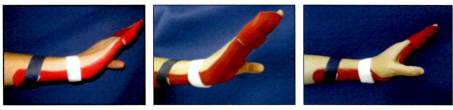

62. Pictured below are several views of the same static splint. This splint would be the **MOST EFFECTIVE** intervention for providing which of the following functions?

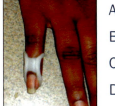

- A. Elongating the finger flexors for a more effective tenodesis grasp
- B. Reducing pain secondary to inflammation of the flexor tendons
- C. Decreasing spasticity secondary to hemiplegia
- D. Stretching the extrinsic finger flexors to reduce soft tissue tightness

63. Pictured below is a splint on the 5th digit of a client's hand. Which option represents the proper purpose for using this type of splint?

- A. To reduce a finger contracture secondary to intrinsic muscle tightness
- B. To manage a boutonnière deformity secondary to an acute jamming injury
- C. To prevent swan neck deformity secondary to subacute rheumatoid arthritis
- D. To prevent a drop finger deformity secondary to an acute mallet finger injury

64. A client is working on a needlework project for a grandchild's birthday, but is having difficulty finishing the project due to low vision from early stage cataracts. The client is scheduled for cataract surgery, but the surgery date is after the grandchild's birthday. Which compensatory technique should the COTA recommend to promote the client's ability to finish the needlework project in time for the birthday?

- A. Advise the client to use high contrast colored thread.
- B. Place the project in an adjustable frame.
- C. Reduce the amount of ambient light in the room.
- D. Provide the client with a lighted, hands-free magnifier.

65. A client sustained a complete T_2 spinal cord injury several months ago. The client is learning compensatory strategies to use for promoting independence and safety during homemaking activities. One of the client's goals is to be able to prepare family meals independently. Which environmental modification would promote progress toward this goal?

- A. Positioning an angled mirror above the stove
- B. Replacing stove knobs with larger handles
- C. Using smaller pans with extended handles
- D. Stirring hot liquids with rubber-coated cooking utensils

66. A client has mild to moderate cognitive decline secondary to dementia. The client has difficulty remembering when to take a prescribed medicine. One of the intervention goals is for the client to independently take medications at the correct dosage times. Which compensatory technique would be **MOST BENEFICIAL** for supporting this goal?

    A. Have a caregiver place medications in a 7-day pill storage container at the beginning of each week.

    B. Advise the client to wear a voice-message alarm pre programmed to activate at specific times of the day.

    C. Teach the client to maintain a medication diary that outlines daily prescription medication requirements and dosage history.

    D. Provide the client with a pocket day-planner that indicates which medications to take each day.

67. Pictured below is an assistive device mounted over a client's stove. What is the **PRIMARY** purpose of this device during stove top cooking?

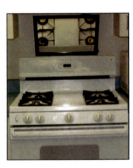

    A. To increase the illumination of contents of the pots by redirecting the kitchen lighting to the stove top

    B. To allow a client with COPD to conserve energy by monitoring contents of pots from a distance

    C. To enable a client who has paraplegia to see the contents of pots when seated in a wheelchair

    D. To provide contrasting visual cues to a client who has low vision.

68. What is the **PRIMARY** purpose for teaching a client who has subacute rheumatoid arthritis to use the assistive device pictured below?

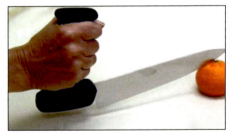

    A. To increase leverage for slicing hard to cut foods

    B. To enable cutting using only one hand

    C. To protect the hand from slipping onto the blade

    D. To reduce deforming forces on the MCP joints

69. A patient sustained a complete C_6 spinal cord injury several weeks ago. One of the intervention goals is to maximize independence with self-feeding. Which assistive device would be **MOST BENEFICIAL** for the patient to use during meals to support this goal?

    A. Switch-operated feeder

    B. Mobile arm support

    C. Tenodesis splint

    D. Wrist cock-up splint

70. A client has symptoms associated with stage 2 Parkinson's disease. One of the intervention goals is for the client to be as independent as possible with self-feeding. Which assistive device would be **MOST BENEFICIAL** for the client to use during meals to support this goal?

   A. Rocker knife

   B. Weighted utensil

   C. Long-handle utensil

   D. Swivel spoon

71. An inpatient sustained an incomplete T_2 spinal cord injury (ASIA C) several weeks ago. One of the intervention goals is for the patient to be independent with wheelchair transfers. The patient is able to transfer without assistive devices from the bed to the wheelchair, but requires moderate assistance when completing transfers from the wheelchair to a standard toilet. What action should the COTA take **NEXT** to support the patient's progress with this transfer skill?

   A. Encourage the patient to use a bedside commode instead of the bathroom toilet.

   B. Teach the patient to use a sliding board transfer to a raised toilet seat.

   C. Complete a manual muscle test to determine the patient's triceps strength.

   D. Evaluate the difference in the height between the wheelchair and the toilet.

72. A client in a home health setting has stage 2 Parkinson's disease. The client had a recent decline in function and is now learning to use a walker for mobility in the home. The COTA is teaching the client how to transport food items in the kitchen using the walker with an attached tray. What information should the COTA include as part of the instructions for minimizing fall risk during this task?

   A. Stand inside the frame of the walker and turn slowly.

   B. Turn the walker to the desired direction then move the legs.

   C. Move the walker to one side and use the counter for support.

   D. Place one hand on the counter and the other on the walker to move it.

73. A patient who had a total hip replacement, anterolateral approach 2 weeks ago wants to lie on the non-affected hip while sleeping. Which adaptation should the patient use when sleeping in this position?

   A. Place a pillow under both feet.

   B. Use an abduction wedge between the legs.

   C. Sleep on memory foam or air mattress.

   D. Flex the affected hip keeping the non-affected leg straight.

74. A COTA is teaching proper bed positioning to the family of a client who has left hemiplegia. What is the **PRIMARY** reason for teaching the family to position the client as indicated in the picture below?

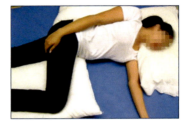

A. To allow unrestricted movement of the unaffected side

B. To prevent a flexor synergy

C. To maintain proper joint alignment

D. To minimize decubitis ulcer formation

75. A COTA working at an assisted living facility is planning to take 8-10 residents on an outing to a restaurant. Several of the residents have hearing impairments. The COTA plans to contact the restaurant in advance of the outing to ask for a table arrangement conducive to the group's socialization. Which table set-up would be **BEST** for this purpose?

A. U-shaped table located close to the kitchen so the residents are comfortable speaking loudly to each other

B. Rectangular table in a busy section of the restaurant so loud talking will not disturb other patrons

C. Round dining table that will comfortably accommodate both the residents and the COTA

D. Several small tables positioned directly under a fluorescent overhead light so residents are able to read and discuss menu options

76. A client who has chronic low back pain is participating in a pain management program. One of the intervention goals is for the client to learn proper body mechanics to use during personal laundry tasks. Which strategy should the COTA teach the client to use for promoting progress toward this goal?

A. Carry one small basket of laundry at a time to the laundry area.

B. Lift one large bundle of clothes from the washer to put into the dryer.

C. Bend forward at the waist while loading clothes into the washer or dryer.

D. Keep the feet shoulder width apart when twisting the torso to place clothes into the dryer.

77. An inpatient in a rehabilitation facility has hemiplegia, moderate short-term memory deficits and impulsiveness secondary to a TBI 3 months ago. Currently, the patient requires moderate cueing for safety during BADL. The patient is preparing for transition to live at home with a spouse as the primary caregiver. One of the discharge goals is to teach the spouse techniques to use at home to support safety when the patient is showering in a stall shower at home. What instructions should the COTA include in the caregiver training to support this goal?

 A. Observe the patient throughout the task to be sure the patient holds onto the grab bar while standing in the shower.

 B. Have the patient sit on a bath stool with suction feet while providing stand-by-assistance throughout the task.

 C. Encourage the patient to use a extended handle reacher and provide hand-over-hand assistance as needed.

 D. Respect the patient's privacy, but remain outside the bathroom door until the patient has turned off the water in the shower.

78. An inpatient has hemiplegia secondary to a recent CVA and is preparing for discharge to live at home with a spouse. The patient has persistent edema of the affected upper extremity despite using proper positioning techniques. One of the intervention goals is to teach the patient methods for managing the edema after discharge. Which action would be **MOST BENEFICIAL** to include as part of the intervention for supporting this goal?

 A. Fabricate a resting hand splint for the patient to wear at all times.

 B. Instruct the patient on how to perform retrograde massage techniques.

 C. Provide the patient with handout instructions for preparing home paraffin baths.

 D. Teach the patient and caregiver to use manual lymphatic treatment techniques.

79. A client who has a substance abuse disorder has been able to maintain employment, but has difficulty managing time, interacting with others, and attending to homemaking activities. What should be the **PRIMARY** focus of the initial intervention for supporting the client's participation in occupation?

 A. To transition the client to a structured group living environment

 B. To promote practical skills for basic personal life management

 C. To encourage the client to participate in leisure activities with friends

 D. To teach the client methods for reducing work-related stressors

80. What should be the **INITIAL** focus of an activity group for inpatients who have been undergoing treatment for major depression?

 A. Completion of a simple craft project

 B. Participation in a short-term familiar task

 C. Interaction in a structured setting

 D. Diversion from the hospital environment

81. A COTA is scheduled to lead a group for young adult clients who have anorexia. One of the objectives of the group is to explore positive behaviors associated with the clients' occupational performance. Which type of activity would be **MOST BENEFICIAL** for supporting this objective?

    A. Incorporate the clients' valued activities into the session.

    B. Select structured craft activities for the clients to complete.

    C. Provide activities based on the clients' self-awareness.

    D. Use a variety of role-playing activities emphasizing body image.

82. A COTA is selecting a group intervention for an inpatient who has paranoid schizophrenia. The patient has transitioned from being self-isolative to tolerating being around several other people at the same time. Which type of group would support the patient's social development?

    A. Parallel

    B. Project

    C. Egocentric-cooperative

    D. Cooperative

83. An adolescent who has a conduct disorder is participating in an OT group to increase socialization skills using a skills acquisition model. While playing a familiar board game, the adolescent loses a turn, becomes frustrated, and demands to play something else. How should the COTA respond to the adolescent's behavior?

    A. Modify the game rules to promote success.

    B. Excuse the adolescent from the activity session.

    C. Encourage the adolescent to complete the activity.

    D. Allow the adolescent to select another activity.

84. A resident of a long term care facility has moderately severe cognitive decline secondary to Alzheimer's disease. Each afternoon when nursing staff change shifts, the resident becomes agitated and attempts to elope from the nursing facility stating, "I need to go back to work." Which action would be **MOST EFFECTIVE** for redirecting the resident's attention and decreasing the risk of elopement?

    A. Have the resident participate in a simple craft activity.

    B. Take the resident outside for a walk around the facility.

    C. Encourage the resident to watch television in the day room.

    D. Begin a reminiscence activity related to something the resident enjoys.

85. An older adult client who has mild macular degeneration is referred to OT. The client is an avid reader and subscribes to several magazines. The client is experiencing progressive difficulty reading the magazines due to the reflective glare from the glossy paper. Which adaptation should the COTA **INITIALLY** recommend to the client for supporting participation in this preferred leisure activity?

    A. Obtain audio and large print books and magazines from a local library.

    B. Subscribe to satellite radio to be able to listen to books and news stories.

    C. Direct the lighting source from behind the shoulder when reading.

    D. Contact publishers for availability of non-glare print issues of the publication.

The following multiple-choice items are samples related to Domain Area 3:

Uphold professional standards and responsibilities to promote quality in practice.

86.   A newly certified COTA recently started working at an inpatient rehabilitation facility. The supervising OTR wants the COTA to assist with administering standardized manual muscle tests as part of patient reevaluations. The COTA has only administered this test to classmates when in school; and received an excellent score on the final laboratory exam. After confirming state licensure regulations permits the COTA to administer standardized tests, what action should the COTA take **NEXT**?

    A. Review class notes on the proper administration procedures for the test.

    B. Ask the OTR to clarify the specific muscles included in the test.

    C. Talk with the OTR about establishing service competency for the test.

    D. Arrange for an OT colleague to observe so inter-rater reliability can be established.

87. A COTA worked in an outpatient hand therapy clinic for the past 5 years. The COTA recently obtained a new job and will be starting work as a COTA in an inpatient neuro-rehabilitation setting. What action should the COTA take as an **INITIAL** step toward developing service competency in the new job?

    A. Arrange a schedule to have close supervision when working with patients.

    B. Provide the OTR with verification of service competent tasks from the previous job.

    C. Learn about clinical protocols by leading a staff discussion on the topic.

    D. Have the supervising OTR review and co-sign each patient contact note.

88. A newly certified COTA recently started a new job in a large rehabilitation clinic. Part of the essential job tasks include fabricating dynamic splints on a routine basis. The COTA received basic splinting instruction in school, yet feels the need for further training. What action would be **MOST BENEFICIAL** for the COTA to take for establishing service competency in this area?

    A. Register to attend an online professional development workshop on splinting.

    B. Arrange for structured mentorship that includes close supervision.

    C. Use a checklist of fabrication tips and techniques when making dynamic splints.

    D. Review school notes and read journal articles about splinting.

89. A COTA is planning an in-service to instruct the nursing staff at a long term care facility about safety techniques to use when transferring patients. What is the **PRIMARY** objective of this type of in-service?

    A. To identify injury risk factors and minimize hazards

    B. To reduce workers' compensation claims within the facility

    C. To comply with legal mandates for staff safety training

    D. To decrease facility liability for job-related injuries

90. An older adult patient is recovering from pneumonia in a subacute setting. The patient has generalized weakness and ambulates independently with a cane in physical therapy sessions. The COTA is scheduled to supervise the patient during self-care sessions. Which risk management technique would be **MOST BENEFICIAL** to use when walking the patient from the bed to the bathroom during the initial session in the patient's room?

    A. Have the patient wear a transfer belt and use a walker.

    B. Ask a caregiver to provide additional stand-by assistance.

    C. Have the patient wear well-fitting non-skid footwear.

    D. Ask the patient to walk with a slow, shuffling gait.

91. A COTA working in a long term psychiatric facility is supervising a craft group for residents who have schizophrenia and are functioning at Allen Cognitive Level 3 (Manual actions). Which action should the COTA ensure takes place prior to the end of the session?

    A. Equipment and supplies used during the session are collected and counted.

    B. Residents wipe the tabletops clean with an antibacterial solution.

    C. Projects are labeled in bold print on a contrasting color background.

    D. Each resident signs an attendance sheet for therapy minutes verification.

92. A COTA is teaching compensatory techniques for facial shaving to a client who has mild choreiform movements of bilateral upper extremities. The COTA wants to be sure standard precautions are followed during this BADL task. Which action should the COTA have the client do as part of this process?

    A. Clean the razor with alcohol after completing the shaving activity.

    B. Practice with an electric shaver borrowed from the OT self-care room.

    C. Bring in a personally-owned electric shaver to use during the session.

    D. Purchase a bag of disposable straight-edge razors.

93. A school-based OTR and COTA are collaborating to evaluate a kindergarten-age student who has autism. Which task can the COTA complete as part of this data gathering process?

    A. Score a sensory integration assessment.

    B. Select developmentally-appropriate assessment tools.

    C. Analyze evaluation results.

    D. Administer a developmental skills checklist.

94. A COTA working in an inpatient rehabilitation clinic is assigned to supervise a newly hired therapy aide. Which information **MUST** the COTA know prior to assigning job tasks to the aide?

    A. State OT practice act guidelines for service provision

    B. Critical demands listed in the aide's job description

    C. Previous experience the aide has had working with patients

    D. Aide's knowledge of occupational therapy interventions

95. A COTA and OTR working in a skilled nursing facility are collaborating to complete an initial intervention plan for a patient who sustained a hip and wrist fracture 5 days ago. Which information **MUST** be included in this patient's documentation to meet Medicare requirements for reimbursement of services?

    A. Pain level and expected changes to strength and ROM by time of discharge

    B. Activities the COTA will be responsible for providing during sessions

    C. Long term functional goals that are medically necessary for the patient

    D. Specific techniques and activities that will be used during sessions

96. A COTA is preparing to write a SOAP progress note for an inpatient who has a complete C_7 spinal cord injury and has been participating in OT for one week to increase independence in upper extremity dressing. The patient is now able to independently sit up in bed and put on a pullover shirt, but still requires caregiver assistance to get the shirt from the closet. Which statement about the patient would be **BEST** to include in the "A" section of the note?

    A. The patient is learning compensatory strategies and is moving towards the long term dressing goal as stated in the initial plan.

    B. The patient will require assistive devices and assistance from a caregiver for most self-care tasks after discharge.

    C. The patient wants to learn how to use additional adaptive devices for lower body dressing and bathing.

    D. The patient scored a "3" (moderate assist) on the dressing section of the Functional Independence Measure (FIM).

97. A patient who had a total knee replacement 3 days ago is being discharged from an acute care facility to an inpatient rehabilitation program. The COTA is contributing outcomes information for the OTR to include in the discharge summary. What information would be **MOST BENEFICIAL** to use for this purpose?

    A. Types of assistive devices used during this phase of recovery

    B. Level of the patient's occupational function prior to hospitalization

    C. Objective information on functional goals achieved

    D. Statements about the patient's participation in goal setting

98. An inpatient is preparing for discharge from an acute mental health setting after undergoing treatment for major depression. The patient will receive follow-up services at a community mental health program. The COTA is contributing outcomes information to the OTR for inclusion in the patient's discharge summary. What information would be **MOST BENEFICIAL** to use for this purpose?

    A. Description of job-related skills the patient used during activities

    B. Patient's functional potential based on current rate of progress

    C. Subjective impressions of the patient's functional independence

    D. Current self-care abilities compared to initial evaluation results

99. Which information should be evident in client contact notes in order to justify the need for additional OT services to a client's insurance company?

    A. Subjective reports of progress in therapy

    B. Progress as it relates to the initial functional goals

    C. Comments on anticipated function at discharge

    D. Rate of progress as compared to other patients

100. A COTA is working in a skilled nursing facility that operates under Medicare regulations. What information **MUST** the COTA document after each intervention session to meet reimbursement requirements of the prospective payment system (PPS)?

    A. Patient's response to specific treatment techniques

    B. Supplies and equipment used during the session

    C. Total number of minutes spent treating the patient

    D. Day and time of the next scheduled treatment session

▶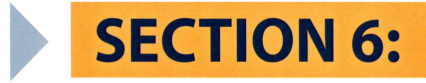

SECTION 6:

Answers, Rationales, and References

Answer Key for the COTA Study Guide Sample Items

Item Number	Key
1	B
2	D
3	A
4	D
5	B
6	D
7	A
8	C
9	B
10	B
11	C
12	B
13	D
14	A
15	A
16	C
17	B
18	A
19	B
20	B
21	C
22	D
23	A
24	D
25	A
26	B
27	D
28	C

Item Number	Key
29	B
30	B
31	B
32	B
33	D
34	A
35	A
36	C
37	D
38	C
39	B
40	A
41	A
42	D
43	C
44	D
45	B
46	B
47	B
48	B
49	A
50	C
51	A
52	A
53	B
54	B
55	D
56	C
57	A
58	A
59	A
60	A
61	D
62	D
63	D
64	D

Item Number	Key
65	A
66	B
67	C
68	D
69	C
70	B
71	D
72	A
73	B
74	C
75	C
76	A
77	B
78	B
79	B
80	B
81	A
82	B
83	C
84	D
85	C
86	C
87	A
88	B
89	A
90	C
91	A
92	C
93	D
94	A
95	C
96	A
97	C
98	D
99	B
100	C

1. *Correct Answer: B*

The initial stage of Parkinson's disease is typically characterized by bradykinesia and incoordination. These symptoms will have the **MOST** impact on the client's ability to self-feed.

Incorrect Answers:

A, C, D. These are not symptoms typically associated with stage 1 Parkinson's Disease.

Reference: Early, M.B. (2013). *Physical Dysfunction Practice Skills for the Occupational Therapy Assistant* (3rd ed.). St. Louis, MO: Elsevier Mosby. Pages 521-524.

2. *Correct Answer: D*

Asking open-ended questions is a non directive method for encouraging the patient's active participation and input in the information gathering process.

Incorrect Answers:

A, B, C. These options are geared towards finding solutions to assist the patient in adapting to retirement, and may be appropriate after first finding out how the patient feels about their retirement.

Reference: Early, M. B. (2009). *Mental Health Concepts and Techniques for the Occupational Therapy Assistant*. (4th ed.). Baltimore, MD: Wolters Kluwer – Lippincott Williams & Wilkins. Pages 38-39.

3. *Correct Answer: A*

Information gathered about the client's vocational interests should be included in the **INITIAL** work readiness evaluation, and used as the basis for further evaluation and intervention planning.

Incorrect Answers:

B, C, D. If deemed necessary, these are tasks the OTR typically completes. They are not appropriate for the COTA to complete as part of the initial data gathering process.

Reference: Early, M. B. (2009). *Mental Health Concepts and Techniques for the Occupational Therapy Assistant*. (4th ed.). Baltimore, MD: Wolters Kluwer – Lippincott Williams & Wilkins. Pages 515-516.

4. *Correct Answer: D*

The **PRIMARY** reason for interviewing the parents is to identify the client's typical performance patterns including safety issues, current skills and abilities, and functional limitations. This information is important for facilitating the client's transition from a supervised home environment to a group home setting.

Incorrect Answers:

A, B, C. Once performance patterns are identified, the other areas can be explored as indicated to promote engagement in occupationally relevant activities.

Reference: Early, M.B. (2013). *Physical Dysfunction Practice Skills for the Occupational Therapy Assistant* (3rd ed.). St. Louis, MO: Elsevier Mosby. Pages 402-403.

5. Correct Answer: B

The **PRIMARY** purpose of this type of analysis is to observe the client performing job tasks in a natural environment. This will provide objective information for determining the impact of the disease in relation to the critical demands of the job.

Incorrect Answers:

A, C. These do not address the physical demands of the job most affected by symptoms of this disease.

D. Special accommodations are mandatory as outlined in the Americans with Disabilities Act.

Reference: Early, M.B. (2013). *Physical Dysfunction Practice Skills for the Occupational Therapy Assistant* (3rd ed.). St. Louis, MO: Elsevier Mosby. Pages 344-345.

6. Correct Answer: D

This type of survey focuses on the clients' perspective about their capacity to engage in purposeful and meaningful activity. Information obtained from the survey is used to develop intervention goals and select intervention activities. It can also be used as a reliable baseline measure for determining progress.

Incorrect Answers:

A, B, C. This type of information is not gathered in an occupational performance measure.

Reference: Early, M.B. (2013). *Physical Dysfunction Practice Skills for the Occupational Therapy Assistant* (3rd ed.). St. Louis, MO: Elsevier Mosby. Pages 82, 84, 592-593.

7. Correct Answer: A

The purpose of the questionnaire is for the clients to identify areas of perceived strengths and weaknesses. This information can be incorporated into the group goal-setting process.

Incorrect Answers:

B. Completing a questionnaire does not facilitate socialization.

C. Responding to this questionnaire does not mean the clients want to address their issues during a group.

D. Evaluating clients' self-assessment skills is not the focus of this type of group.

Reference: Early, M. B. (2009). *Mental Health Concepts and Techniques for the Occupational Therapy Assistant*. (4th ed.). Baltimore, MD: Wolters Kluwer – Lippincott Williams & Wilkins. Pages 448-449,543.

8. Correct Answer: C

Tactile gnosis is the ability to recognize familiar objects by touch with vision occluded. A client with tactile agnosia would not be able to find a key in a pocket since the client would not be able to distinguish the object characteristics without the aid of visual cues.

Incorrect Answers:

A, B, D. The vision is typically not occluded during these functional tasks. Tactile agnosia would not be as evident since the client would be able to complete the task by using visual cues.

Reference: Early, M. B. (2009). *Mental Health Concepts and Techniques for the Occupational Therapy Assistant.* (4th ed.). Baltimore, MD: Wolters Kluwer – Lippincott Williams & Wilkins. Page 461.

9. Correct Answer: B

When administrating a standardized assessment, the established administration procedures must be strictly followed. If the protocols are not followed, the assessment results are not reliable.

Incorrect Answers:

A, C, D. When administering a standardized assessment, the OT practitioner may not alter or modify the test protocols, as this would alter the reliability of the assessment.

Reference: Early, M.B. (2013). *Physical Dysfunction Practice Skills for the Occupational Therapy Assistant* (3rd ed.). St. Louis, MO: Elsevier Mosby. Page 60.

10. Correct Answer: B

Assessment of the patient's BADL routines and current functional skill level is required **FIRST** to determine the durable medical equipment, assistive devices and instructions necessary to promote bathing independence.

Incorrect Answers:

A, D. Determining the patient's ability to use adaptive equipment and teaching adaptive bathing techniques should begin after obtaining information about current self-care routines and abilities.

C. Obtaining general information about the home set-up can be done as part of the initial interview. More detailed information should be obtained after determining the client's current functional skill level and typical BADL routines.

Reference: Padilla, R. L., Byers-Connon, S., Lohman, H. (2012). *Occupational Therapy with Elders: Strategies for the COTA.* (3rd ed.). St. Louis, MO: Elsevier Mosby. Pages 264-265.

Early, M.B. (2013). *Physical Dysfunction Practice Skills for the Occupational Therapy Assistant* (3rd ed.). St. Louis, MO: Elsevier Mosby. Pages 58-59.

11. Correct Answer: C

The Individual's with Disabilities Education Act (IDEA) mandates that eligibility requirements for IEP services are based on the student's classroom needs and performance in relation to curriculum-based objectives.

Incorrect Answers:

A. A physician referral is typically not necessary to initiate school-based OT intervention.

B. Eligibility for IEP services cannot be based solely on standardized test scores and a documented disability.

D. These are not primary factors for determining a student's eligibility for school-based IEP services

Reference: Solomon, J. W., O'Brien, J. C. (2011). *Pediatric Skills for Occupational Therapy Assistants*. (3rd ed.). St. Louis, MO: Elsevier Mosby. Pages 46-47.

12. Correct Answer: B

Information about the patient's cultural values should be used to guide intervention plans and activities.

Incorrect Answers:

A. This option may result in false assumptions and stereotypical bias regarding the patient's culture

C. This assumes the patient does not speak English and is not the **INITIAL** action the COTA should take in this situation.

D. Many standardized OT evaluation tools do not have cross-cultural validity. Therefore, the norms cannot be used to report evaluation results.

Reference: Early, M.B. (2013). *Physical Dysfunction Practice Skills for the Occupational Therapy Assistant* (3rd ed.). St. Louis, MO: Elsevier Mosby. Pages 181-182.

13. Correct Answer: D

All clients have the right to refuse treatment; however, to maintain participation in therapy the COTA should offer the client an alternate choice of activity.

Incorrect Answers:

A. The spiritual diversity and rights of all group participants must be acknowledged and respected.

B, C. The client has a right to refuse participation in the task due to religious reasons. It is not necessary for the client to discuss this with a counselor or to explore reasons for a conflict.

Reference: Sladyk K., Jacobs K., MacRae, N. (2010). *Occupational Therapy Essentials for Clinical Competence*. Thorofare, NJ: SLACK Inc. Page 39, 210.

14. *Correct Answer: A*

The COTA should gather information about the client's values, routines, habits and expectations. When teaching homemaking skills the COTA should respect and support the client 's cultural preferences.

Incorrect Answers: A

B, D. These do not take into account the client's established homemaking habits and routines.

C. The COTA needs to first establish if this activity respects the client's culture and values before incorporating it into a treatment session.

Reference: Early, M. B. (2009). *Mental Health Concepts and Techniques for the Occupational Therapy Assistant*. (4th ed.). Baltimore, MD: Wolters Kluwer – Lippincott Williams & Wilkins. Pages 244, 500.

15. *Correct Answer: A*

The physician needs to know that the client is noncompliant. Abruptly stopping medication can result in physical and psychological consequences.

Incorrect Answers:

B. The client's family cannot be notified unless the client has signed a consent form.

C. This may be an option only after contacting the physician and discussing the option with the OTR.

D. A behavioral contract for medication compliance should be done under the direction of the physician.

Reference: Early, M. B. (2009). *Mental Health Concepts and Techniques for the Occupational Therapy Assistant*. (4th ed.). Baltimore, MD: Wolters Kluwer – Lippincott Williams &Wilkins. Pages 493-494.

16. *Correct Answer: C*

The COTA should **INITIALLY** stop the activity for the day and alert the charge nurse of the patient's symptoms. Extreme fatigue can trigger an exacerbation of multiple sclerosis.

Incorrect Answers:

A, D. Client's should use energy conservation and work simplification as fatigue management techniques to minimize the onset of fatigue.

B. This may help with activity completion, but does manage the patient's fatigue for reducing the risk of relapse.

Reference: Early, M.B. (2013). *Physical Dysfunction Practice Skills for the Occupational Therapy Assistant* (3rd ed.). St. Louis, MO: Elsevier Mosby. Pages 517-519.

17. Correct Answer: B

The COTA should **INITIALLY** discuss with the client any changes in behavior that may have an impact on the client's intervention goals or overall outcomes.

Incorrect Answers:

A, C, D. These options may be indicated after discussing the observations and concerns with the client.

Reference: Early, M.B. (2013). *Physical Dysfunction Practice Skills for the Occupational Therapy Assistant* (3rd ed.). St. Louis, MO: Elsevier Mosby. Pages 62-63, 67.

18. Correct Answer: A

These symptoms are consistent with autonomic dysreflexia which is life-threatening. The **INITIAL** action the COTA should take is to obtain emergency medical assistance.

Incorrect Answers:

B. This is not the **INITIAL** action the COTA should take in this life-threatening situation.

C. The COTA should stop the activity but should seek medical assistance first; not wait for vital signs to stabilize.

D. This action is contraindicated for symptoms associated with autonomic dysreflexia.

Reference: Early, M.B. (2013). *Physical Dysfunction Practice Skills for the Occupational Therapy Assistant* (3rd ed.). St. Louis, MO: Elsevier Mosby. Page 539.

19. Correct Answer: B

The COTA should **INITIALLY** consider the factors that contributed to the combative behaviors. This allows the COTA to identify effective solutions for de-escalating the agitation.

Incorrect Answers:

A. This should not be the **INITIAL** action for the COTA to take.

C. This may increase the resident's agitation.

D. Altering the resident's typical routines may result in increased agitation and confusion. Additionally, afternoons are typically associated with symptoms of sun-downing.

Reference: Padilla, R. L., Byers-Connon, S., Lohman, H. (2012). *Occupational Therapy with Elders: Strategies for the COTA.* (3rd ed.). St. Louis, MO: Elsevier Mosby. Pages 279-280.

20. Correct Answer: B

Intense pain or an unpleasant experience may cause a temporary autonomic vasovagal response. As a result the heart rate and blood pressure drop, which reduces the blood flow to the brain. This results in a feeling of warmth, light-headedness, dimming vision and hearing, and even fainting (vasovagal syncope). The client must be quickly reclined with the legs elevated in order for their blood pressure to return to normal.

Incorrect Answers:

A, D. This will not assist with elevating the client's blood pressure.

C. This is likely to further contribute to the client's lowering blood pressure.

Reference: Early, M.B. (2013). *Physical Dysfunction Practice Skills for the Occupational Therapy Assistant* (3rd ed.). St. Louis, MO: Elsevier Mosby. Page 47.

21. Correct Answer: C

From the list provided, this set of homemaking tasks requires the **GREATEST** amount of bilateral shoulder flexion and elbow extension.

Incorrect Answers:

A, B, D. These tasks do not require as much shoulder flexion and elbow extension as folding sheets and hanging towels on a clothesline.

Reference: Early, M.B. (2013). *Physical Dysfunction Practice Skills for the Occupational Therapy Assistant* (3rd ed.). St. Louis, MO: Elsevier Mosby. Pages 119-123, 209-210.

22. Correct Answer: D

This activity promotes goal attainment through the use of meaningful tasks that have an inherent purpose.

Incorrect Answers:

A, B. Although simulated and isometric activities alone may assist with goal attainment, they are not the primary focus of the activity described.

C. Although cleanliness in the home may be achieved during this activity, the goal of the activity is to increase active shoulder flexion through purposeful activity.

Reference: Early, M.B. (2013). *Physical Dysfunction Practice Skills for the Occupational Therapy Assistant* (3rd ed.). St. Louis, MO: Elsevier Mosby. Pages 207-208.

23. Correct Answer: A

Low vision can impact residents' functional performance in a variety of ways. It is important to identify individual needs prior to implementing new procedures or making environmental changes.

Incorrect Answers:

B, C, D. These are generic modifications and are not based on specific needs of the individual residents.

Reference: Padilla, R. L., Byers-Connon, S., Lohman, H. (2012). *Occupational Therapy with Elders: Strategie. for the COTA.* (3rd ed.). St. Louis, MO: Elsevier Mosby, Inc. Page 225.

Sladyk K., Jacobs K., MacRae N. (2010). *Occupational Therapy Essentials for Clinical Competence.* Thorofare, NJ: SLACK Inc. Page 239.

24. Correct Answer: D

Based on the patient's current level of functioning, the patient's private room is **MOST CONDUCIVE** for promoting progress because it provides the least distractions and is most familiar to the patient.

Incorrect Answers:

A. A quiet area in the rehabilitation department may still have multiple distractions. The patient's unfamiliarity with this area may further confuse the patient.

B. This environment may be over-stimulating for the patient and may increase the patient's agitatio and confusion.

C. Seated on a tub bench is not optimal for promoting the patient's lower body dressing success.

Reference: Early, M.B. (2013). *Physical Dysfunction Practice Skills for the Occupational Therapy Assistant* (3rd ed.). St. Louis, MO: Elsevier Mosby. Page 509.

25. Correct Answer: A

Short term goals must be objective, achievable, measurable, and contain a time frame for completion. For a patient in the recovery phase of Guillain-Barré syndrome short term goals should be carefully graded to prevent relapse.

Incorrect Answers:

B. Use of proper body mechanics is important, but the statement does not reflect a short term goal that is achievable during the next phase of rehabilitation.

C. This goal does not contain a timeframe for completion.

D. This is too general for a short term goal and does not reflect a functional task.

Reference: Early, M.B. (2013). *Physical Dysfunction Practice Skills for the Occupational Therapy Assistant* (3rd ed.). St. Louis, MO: Elsevier Mosby. Pages 80, 84, 72-73, 560-561.

Sladyk, K., Jacobs, K., MacRae N. (2010). *Occupational Therapy Essentials for Clinical Competence.* Thorofare, NJ: SLACK Inc. Page 359.

26. *Correct Answer: B*

The COTA should collaborate with the OTR prior to changing the intervention plan or discontinuing OT services.

Incorrect Answers:

A, C, D. Discontinuing OT, re-evaluating the client, or advising the client not to attend a group are decisions the OTR should make with input from the COTA.

Reference: Early, M. B. (2009). *Mental Health Concepts and Techniques for the Occupational Therapy Assistant.* (4th ed.). Baltimore, MD: Wolters Kluwer – Lippincott Williams & Wilkins. Page 452.

27. *Correct Answer: D*

The COTA may identify the need for change to the treatment process. Any changes made to the treatment plan and goals should be done in collaboration with the OTR.

Incorrect Answers:

A. The OTR is responsible for revising the intervention plan.

B. The COTA must discuss the patient's progress with the OTR prior to administering a standardized assessment.

C. It is not necessary for the COTA to discuss this progress with the physician prior to the next BADL session.

Reference: Early, M.B. (2013). *Physical Dysfunction Practice Skills for the Occupational Therapy Assistant* (3rd ed.). St. Louis, MO: Elsevier Mosby. Pages 54-55, 72.

28. *Correct Answer: C*

In a school-based setting, it is **MOST IMPORTANT** to communicate the student's progress related to curriculum-based school activities.

Incorrect Answers:

A. This is typically not the focus of a reevaluation for a student at this grade level.

B. Motor performance of the student compared to typically developing children does not provide the information related to the student's functional goals in a school setting.

D. Leisure skill development should not be the focus of school-based services.

Reference: Solomon, J. W., O'Brien, J. C. (2011). *Pediatric Skills for Occupational Therapy Assistants.* (3rd ed.). St. Louis, MO: Elsevier Mosby. Pages 53-55.

29. Correct Answer: B

The primary role of the COTA is to make recommendations about environmental adaptations to enable the resident to access toilet facilities safely and independently. In addition, the COTA can advise on clothing adaptations and activities to improve the efficiency of managing clothing during toilet activities.

Incorrect Answers:

A, C, D. The COTA may contribute to discussions on these topics, but these tasks are primarily completed by other members of the multidisciplinary team.

Reference: Padilla, R. L., Byers-Connon, S., Lohman, H. (2012). *Occupational Therapy with Elders: Strategie for the COTA*. (3rd ed.). St. Louis, MO: Elsevier Mosby. Page 245.

30. Correct Answer: B

Based on scope of practice guidelines, the COTA would be responsible for reporting students progress during school-related activities.

Incorrect Answers:

A. Information presented at the IEP must be related to curriculum-based activities and progress.

C. The OTR typically considers these standardized assessment scores for intervention planning. The COTA is not typically expected to report these scores during IEP reviews.

D. These skills are typically addressed by the speech and language pathologist.

Reference: Solomon, J. W., O'Brien, J. C. (2011). *Pediatric Skills for Occupational Therapy Assistants*. (3rd ed.). St. Louis, MO: Elsevier Mosby. Pages 53-54.

31. Correct Answer: B

The client's ability to follow through with a self-directed program impacts functional outcomes and is **MOST IMPORTANT** to consider.

Incorrect Answers:

A. Having a detailed understanding of the home program rationale is not essential. Although the client should have a general idea that the program is a means to a functional goal.

C. Depending on the type of neurobehavioral deficit, the client may have difficulty verbalizing steps of the program, or the client may be able to verbalize the steps but may not be able to complete the steps independently.

D. Family support is useful information to consider when providing a home exercise program, but is not as important; especially if the client can demonstrate independent follow-through of the home program.

Reference: Early, M.B. (2013). *Physical Dysfunction Practice Skills for the Occupational Therapy Assistant* (3rd ed.). St. Louis, MO: Elsevier Mosby. Pages 181-182.

32. *Correct Answer: B*

> Providing the family with guidance and support for promoting the patient's function at home is an important role of the COTA in the discharge planning process.

Incorrect Answers:

> A. The patient's family may choose to have an aide assist in the care or obtain respite care; however, the COTA should provide the family with behavioral strategies for supporting the patient's function at home – especially since the family will be responsible for assisting the patient when aide services are not in the home.

> C. Based on the stage of cognitive decline, the patient would have difficulty learning how to use assistive devices and new ways for completing BADL.

> D. This is not within the scope of practice for the COTA.

> **Reference:** Early, M.B. (2013). *Physical Dysfunction Practice Skills for the Occupational Therapy Assistant* (3rd ed.). St. Louis, MO: Elsevier Mosby. Pages 528-529.

33. *Correct Answer: D*

> Amyotrophic lateral sclerosis is a progressive degenerative neuromuscular disease. Disease progression is rapid resulting in significant mobility deficits and eventual paralysis. Information about durable medical equipment (DME) needs for the home environment is **MOST IMPORTANT** given the patient's goal to live at home as long as possible.

Incorrect Answers:

> A. Discussing the patient's prior vocational and leisure history does not assist the patient's goal to live at home as long as possible. It is more important to address DME needs due to the recent decline in function.

> B. It is unnecessary to inform the team of these specific measurements.

> C. This is not appropriate since the patient's goal is to reside at home for as long as possible.

> **Reference:** Early, M.B. (2013). *Physical Dysfunction Practice Skills for the Occupational Therapy Assistant* (3rd ed.). St. Louis, MO: Elsevier Mosby. Pages 55, 68, 525-527.

34. *Correct Answer: A*

> The COTA should collaborate with the patient and relevant others in order to prioritize the patient's needs.

Incorrect Answers:

> B, C. Collaboration with the patient and family should be done prior to making changes or recommending changes to the apartment manager.

> D. The OTR or the physical therapist would be responsible for assessing the patient's ability to ambulate using a walker.

> **Reference:** Early, M.B. (2013). *Physical Dysfunction Practice Skills for the Occupational Therapy Assistant* (3rd ed.). St. Louis, MO: Elsevier Mosby. Pages 243-248.

35. Correct Answer: A

The COTA should **INITIALLY** collaborate with the client regarding the barriers to participation in OT and the potential solutions.

Incorrect Answers:

B, D. Providing an independent home program and a monthly reevaluation are less effective than active participation in OT at this stage of the client's rehabilitation.

C. The client does not meet the eligibility requirements for home health services since the client is not "home bound".

Reference: Early, M.B. (2013). *Physical Dysfunction Practice Skills for the Occupational Therapy Assistant* (3rd ed.). St. Louis, MO: Elsevier Mosby. Pages 31-32.

36. Correct Answer: C

Effective caregiver education is a central component of care. In-service education would provide the staff with more insight about the benefits and proper use of the equipment for the residents' specific needs.

Incorrect Answers:

A. This is not the **MOST BENEFICIAL** option for supporting the residents' needs or the aides motivation for positive change.

B. This may not be possible based on the residents' physical and cognitive condition.

D. Although this may be helpful in the short-term, an in-service would provide the staff with more insight about the benefits of the equipment for the residents' specific needs.

Reference: Padilla, R. L., Byers-Connon, S., Lohman, H. (2012). *Occupational Therapy with Elders: Strategies for the COTA.* (3rd ed.). St. Louis, MO: Elsevier Mosby. Page 147.

37. Correct Answer: D

It is **MOST IMPORTANT** to educate employees about work-related risk factors. Of the options presented, this has the greatest impact on preventing injuries – which is the purpose of the in-service.

Incorrect Answers:

A, C. This information is beneficial to the company management, but has relatively little meaning to the general employee population and is not the purpose of the in-service.

B. This information should not be provided unless indicated as part of an intervention plan for rehabilitation of a specific injury.

Reference: Early, M.B. (2013). *Physical Dysfunction Practice Skills for the Occupational Therapy Assistant* (3rd ed.). St. Louis, MO: Elsevier Mosby. Pages 346-349.

38. Correct Answer: C

The emphasis for clients attending a substance abuse program is on improving function and providing skill development.

Incorrect Answers:

A. Part of relapse prevention includes recognizing triggers that lead to misuse.

B, D. These choices are not a primary role of the COTA in this type of program development process.

Reference: Early, M. B. (2009). *Mental Health Concepts and Techniques for the Occupational Therapy Assistant.* (4th ed.). Baltimore, MD: Wolters Kluwer – Lippincott Williams & Wilkins. Page 161.

39. Correct Answer: B

An interactive discussion is not only informative, but can be tailored to the participants' interests and concerns.

Incorrect Answers:

A. The goal of the presentation is to communicate the role of occupational therapy in assisting individuals who have systemic lupus. Providing information about specific assessments would be more appropriate for an audience of healthcare team members.

C, D. Providing a simulation of a therapy session or demonstrating an exercise program does not provide a broad perspective about the services that OT has to offer for individuals who have this disease. Additionally, these do not address the specific concerns of the attendees.

Reference: Early, M.B. (2013). *Physical Dysfunction Practice Skills for the Occupational Therapy Assistant* (3rd ed.). St. Louis, MO: Elsevier Mosby. Pages 181-184, 574-575.

40. Correct Answer: A

This activity would be **MOST BENEFICIAL** for promoting bilateral use of the upper extremities at a developmentally appropriate level.

Incorrect Answers:

B, C, D. These are play activities for typically developing children between the ages of 4 and 8 years of age.

Reference: Solomon, J. W., O'Brien, J. C. (2011). *Pediatric Skills for Occupational Therapy Assistants.* (3rd ed.). St. Louis, MO: Elsevier Mosby. Pages 122-123.

41. Correct Answer: A

Of the choices provided, this is the only activity that promotes bilateral hand use.

Incorrect Answers:

B, C, D. These answers are most often performed unilaterally. Therefore, they would not be the **MOST BENEFICIAL** activities for promoting bilateral hand-use.

Reference: Solomon, J. W., O'Brien, J. C. (2011). *Pediatric Skills for Occupational Therapy Assistants.* (3rd ed.). St. Louis, MO: Elsevier Mosby. Page 464.

42. Correct Answer: D

This activity encourages fine motor control and isolated thumb and finger prehension to improve pencil grasp development.

Incorrect Answers:

A. This activity would not be effective for developing the fine motor control needed for a mature pencil grasp.

B, C. Since the student has good proximal control, these activities would not be as effective as stringing beads for developing the fine motor or isolated finger movement patterns to promote a more mature pencil grasp.

Reference: Solomon, J. W., O'Brien, J. C. (2011). *Pediatric Skills for Occupational Therapy Assistants*. (3rd ed.). St. Louis, MO: Elsevier Mosby. Page 429.

43. Correct Answer: C

Creating rhymes about school assignments is **MOST BENEFICIAL** for helping the student to process, remember, and recall information through the use of language cues.

Incorrect Answers:

A, B, D. These activities would not be **MOST BENEFICIAL** for promoting directionality for a student who is an auditory learner.

Reference: Solomon, J. W., O'Brien, J. C. (2011). *Pediatric Skills for Occupational Therapy Assistants*. (3rd ed.). St. Louis, MO: Elsevier Mosby. Page 433.

44. Correct Answer: D

This child must **INITIALLY** learn to integrate and process sensory input as a precursor to learning Braille.

Incorrect Answers:

A. This option is contraindicated as an initial intervention for tactile defensiveness.

B, C. These options do not address sensory processing deficits related to tactile defensiveness.

Reference: Solomon, J. W., O'Brien, J. C. (2011). *Pediatric Skills for Occupational Therapy Assistants*. (3rd ed.). St. Louis, MO: Elsevier Mosby. Pages 220-221.

45. Correct Answer: B

This tactile media provides proprioceptive input that will help the student learn the motor patterns necessary for improving handwriting skills.

Incorrect Answers:

A, C, D. These activities do not provide the proprioceptive input needed to plan the motor movements for writing.

Reference: Solomon, J. W., O'Brien, J. C. (2011). *Pediatric Skills for Occupational Therapy Assistants*. (3rd ed.). St. Louis, MO: Elsevier Mosby. Pages 431-433.

46. Correct Answer: B

This choice is an inhibitory technique and is therefore **MOST EFFECTIVE** for reducing muscle tone.

Incorrect Answers:

A, C, D. These are facilitation techniques used to increase muscle tone.

Reference: Solomon, J. W., O'Brien, J. C. (2011). *Pediatric Skills for Occupational Therapy Assistants*. (3rd ed.). St. Louis, MO: Elsevier Mosby. Page 337.

47. Correct Answer: B

Blowing soap bubbles is a motivating age-appropriate play activity that promotes lip closure and oral motor control.

Incorrect Answers:

A. Drinking thin liquids from this type of cup would result in spillage and would not be **MOST BENEFICIAL** to include as part of the child's initial intervention.

C, D. These tasks are developmentally inappropriate.

Reference: Delany, J.V., Pendzick, M.J. (2009). *Working with Children and Adolescents: A Guide for the Occupational Therapy Assistant*. Upper Saddle River, N.J.: Pearson Prentice Hall. Pages 226-229.

48. Correct Answer: B

Flexion of the affected extremities and trunk is **MOST EFFECTIVE** for inhibiting extensor tone. Facing the student away from the caregiver enables the caregiver to position the student using good body mechanics.

Incorrect Answers:

A, C. These positions contribute to increased extensor tone during the transfer.

D. Positioning the student in this manner does not provide adequate hip and knee flexion to inhibit extensor tone.

Reference: Solomon, J. W., O'Brien, J. C. (2011). *Pediatric Skills for Occupational Therapy Assistants*. (3rd ed.). St. Louis, MO: Elsevier Mosby. Pages 325-331.

49. Correct Answer: A

This position increases proximal stability for better hand and wrist movement during writing tasks.

Incorrect Answers:

B, C, D. These are not compensatory strategies for enhancing proximal stability during a handwriting task.

Reference: Case-Smith, J. & O'Brien, J.C. (2010). *Occupational Therapy for Children*. (6th ed.). St. Louis, MO: Elsevier Mosby. Pages 569-570.

Solomon, J. W., O'Brien, J. C. (2011). *Pediatric Skills for Occupational Therapy Assistants*. (3rd ed.). St. Louis, MO: Elsevier Mosby. Pages 427-429.

50. Correct Answer: C

Sitting in front of the child and slightly below the child's eye level inhibits the persistent primitive reflexes which interfere with bilateral hand skills and hand to mouth movements.

Incorrect Answers:

A, B, D. These positions may trigger the persistent primitive reflexes which interfere with independent movement of the head and extremities.

Reference: DeLany, J.V., Pendzick M.J. (2009).*Working with Children and Adolescents: A Guide for the Occupational Therapy Assistant*. Upper Saddle River, N.J.: Pearson Prentice Hall. Pages 229, 476

51. Correct Answer: A

Clients with a complete spinal cord injury at this level typically have upper extremity ROM and strength for manual wheelchair propulsion of a lightweight folding wheelchair with modified rims.

Incorrect Answers:

B. This type of wheelchair would be more useful for a higher level spinal cord injury.

C. This mobility option does not allow navigation on all indoor surface and outdoor terrain.

D. This type of wheelchair is too heavy and does not provide the needed rim modification for manual propulsion.

Reference: Early, M.B. (2013). *Physical Dysfunction Practice Skills for the Occupational Therapy Assistant* (3rd ed.). St. Louis, MO: Elsevier Mosby. Pages 545-549.

52. Correct Answer: A

Head movements to either side can trigger the asymmetrical tonic neck reflex (ATNR). Placing the paint in front of the student is **MOST EFFECTIVE** for minimizing side-to-side head movements.

Incorrect Answers:

B. Adding weight does not inhibit the ATNR.

C, D. The student would still have to reach for the paint; triggering the ATNR.

Reference: Solomon, J. W., O'Brien, J. C. (2011). *Pediatric Skills for Occupational Therapy Assistants*. (3rd ed.). St. Louis, MO: Elsevier Mosby. Pages 88-91, 306-307, 313-314.

53. Correct Answer: B

MCP joint ulnar drift is a characteristic deformity associated with rheumatoid arthritis. To protect the MCP joints, clients who have rheumatoid arthritis should avoid movements that place these joints in ulnar deviation.

Incorrect Answers:

A, C, D. Wrist extension, wrist ulnar deviation, and composite finger extension are not deforming forces inherent to the activities that seem to cause pain for this client.

Reference: Early, M.B. (2013). *Physical Dysfunction Practice Skills for the Occupational Therapy Assistant* (3rd ed.). St. Louis, MO: Elsevier Mosby. Pages 193-194, 573-574, 581-585.

54. *Correct Answer: B*

Homonymous hemianopsia typically results after a CVA of the posterior cerebral artery. Hemianopsia affects the visual field of both eyes and results in a neglect or inattention to a specific visual space.

Incorrect Answers:

A. A client who has figure-ground deficits has difficulty distinguishing a specific feature from the background (e.g., how many cookies are on each pan).

C. Reduced depth perception may affect a client's ability to judge distance. This would impact the ability to place a cookie tray on the oven rack, but would not affect a specific field of vision.

D. Laterality deficits impair a client's ability to distinguish between right and left sides, but do not result in avoiding one side of the environment.

Reference: Early, M.B. (2013). *Physical Dysfunction Practice Skills for the Occupational Therapy Assistant* (3rd ed.). St. Louis, MO: Elsevier Mosby. Pages 442-443.

55. *Correct Answer: D*

Decreased platelet levels can result in an increased risk of prolonged bleeding if the patient is cut. Activities requiring sharp tools present a risk management issue and are not advisable for the patient to use.

Incorrect Answers:

A, B, C. There are no special precautions associated with these materials for patients who have this condition.

Reference: Early, M.B. (2013). *Physical Dysfunction Practice Skills for the Occupational Therapy Assistant* (3rd ed.). St. Louis, MO: Elsevier Mosby. Page 691.

56. *Correct Answer: C*

This activity is **MOST BENEFICIAL** because it involves working on fine motor skills using an activity that is meaningful and important to the client.

Incorrect Answers:

A, B. The task that is important to the client is playing the piano. These choices may improve strength and fine motor control, but do not incorporate the client's valued activity.

D. This does not directly support the client's goal of being able to resume playing the piano.

Reference: Early, M.B. (2013). *Physical Dysfunction Practice Skills for the Occupational Therapy Assistant* (3rd ed.). St. Louis, MO: Elsevier Mosby. Pages 377-378.

57. Correct Answer: A

It is **MOST IMPORTANT** to reinforce the principles of energy conservation by making sure the supplies are available and within easy reach.

Incorrect Answers:

B, D. Patients who have COPD should be seated during self-care tasks. Placing a chair outside of the bathroom is not helpful.

C. Using spray deodorants and powders is contraindicated for patients who have breathing difficulties secondary to COPD.

Reference: Padilla, R. L., Byers-Connon, S., Lohman, H. (2012). *Occupational Therapy with Elders: Strategie* *for the COTA*. (3rd ed.). St. Louis, MO: Elsevier Mosby. Pages 324-325.

58. Correct Answer: A

Symptoms of decreased visual acuity include inability to see objects clearly, difficulty distinguishing visual details and difficulty discriminating contrast and colors. Labeling food items using large print labels and high-contrast colors would be **MOST BENEFICIAL** for enabling clients with decreased visual acuity use the remaining vision to enhance functional performance.

Incorrect Answers:

B. Fluorescent bulbs produce glare or shadows on work surfaces that may further interfere with visual acuity.

C. Keeping items on the counter top may make these items more accessible; however, would not compensate for a visual acuity deficit.

D. Glass panels on cabinet doors may produce reflective glare which further interferes with visual acuity.

Reference: Early, M.B. (2013). *Physical Dysfunction Practice Skills for the Occupational Therapy Assistant* (3rd ed.). St. Louis, MO: Elsevier Mosby. Page 441.

59. Correct Answer: A

COPD typically causes dyspnea, shortness of breath and fatigue. Learning energy conservation techniques during the **INITIAL** phase of rehabilitation will promote the client's functional performance within the limitations of the COPD symptoms.

Incorrect Answers:

B, C, D. These options may be considered later in the intervention process based on the client's needs and goals.

Reference: Early, M.B. (2013). *Physical Dysfunction Practice Skills for the Occupational Therapy Assistant* (3rd ed.). St. Louis, MO: Elsevier Mosby. Pages 682-687.

60. *Correct Answer: A*

Using breathing technique during exertion would be **MOST EFFECTIVE** for the client to use for reducing demands on the lungs and cardiovascular system.

Incorrect Answers:

B, C, D. These techniques are not effective for managing the symptoms of COPD.

Reference: Early, M.B. (2013). *Physical Dysfunction Practice Skills for the Occupational Therapy Assistant* (3rd ed.). St. Louis, MO: Elsevier Mosby. Pages 686-687.

61. *Correct Answer: D*

Application of lotion to areas of dry skin and compression wrapping will help reduce the edema and create skin softening and reduce the edema.

Incorrect Answers:

A. This may increase the edema during this phase of healing.

B. Pulsed ultrasound would be more effective than continuous wave low intensity ultrasound.

C. Low intensity vibration may be beneficial during the later phases of healing.

Reference: Early, M.B. (2013). *Physical Dysfunction Practice Skills for the Occupational Therapy Assistant* (3rd ed.). St. Louis, MO: Elsevier Mosby. Page 601.

Radomski, M.V., Trombly Latham C.A. (2008). *Occupational Therapy for Physical Dysfunction* (6th ed.). Baltimore, MD: Wolters Kluwer – Lippincott Williams & Wilkins. Page 1142.

62. *Correct Answer: D*

The extrinsic finger flexors cross multiple joints. Positioning the wrist and fingers in composite extension will help to stretch tight extrinsic finger flexors.

Incorrect Answers:

A. Stretching the extrinsic finger flexors is contraindicated for establishing an effective tenodesis grasp.

B. This place tension on the finger flexors and will increase pain if the tendons are inflamed.

C. This position will not decrease spasticity.

Reference: Cooper, C. (2007). *Fundamentals of Hand Therapy*. St. Louis, MO: Elsevier Mosby. Pages 444-445.

Keough, J.L., Sain, S.J., Roller, C.L. (2012). *Kinesiology for the Occupational Therapy Assistant: Essential Components of Function and Movement*. Thorofare, N.J.: SLACK, Inc. Pages 73-74, 274-275.

63. Correct Answer: D

A mallet finger injury results in drop finger deformity (DIP joint flexion) secondary to a rupture of the terminal portion of the finger extensor. Conservative treatment includes continuous immobilization of the DIP joint in full extension or hyperextension while the tendon heals.

Incorrect Answers:

A. Intrinsic muscles do not effect the DIP joint.

B. This deformity results in PIP joint flexion and DIP joint hyperextension. The appropriate splint should focus on aligning both joints.

C. This deformity results in PIP joint hyperextension and DIP joint flexion. The appropriate splint should focus on aligning both joints.

Reference: Coppard, B.M., Lohman, H.M. (2007). *Splinting: A Clinical Reasoning & Problem-Solving Approach*. St. Louis, MO: Elsevier Mosby. Pages 444-445. Pages 259-260.

Keough, J.L., Sain, S.J., Roller, C.L. (2012). *Kinesiology for the Occupational Therapy Assistant: Essential Components of Function and Movement*. Thorofare, N.J.: SLACK, Inc. Pages 263-264.

64. Correct Answer: D

In the early stage of cataract development, a magnifier can be a helpful device to compensate for inadequate visual acuity.

Incorrect Answers:

A. Changing the type of thread is not realistic, since the client has already started the project.

B. This does not impact the client's ability to see the work area.

C. This would not improve the clarity of the blurred vision for completing this project.

Reference: Padilla, R. L., Byers-Connon, S., Lohman, H. (2012). *Occupational Therapy with Elders: Strategies for the COTA*. (3rd ed.). St. Louis, MO: Elsevier Mosby. Pages 215, 221-222.

65. Correct Answer: A

A client who has a complete T_2 spinal cord injury depends on a wheelchair for mobility. When preparing meals while seated in a wheelchair, it is difficult to see contents of pots and pans on the stove top. Placing a mirror over the stove enables the client to see food as it is cooking, and to determine the temperature from observation.

Incorrect Answers:

B, D. Paraplegia does not impair clients' manual dexterity or upper extremity strength.

C. Smaller pans are more manageable to lift; however, reaching across burners is not as safe as using the front burners on the stove.

Reference: Early, M.B. (2013). *Physical Dysfunction Practice Skills for the Occupational Therapy Assistant* (3rd ed.). St. Louis, MO: Elsevier Mosby. Pages 267-269, 550.

66. *Correct Answer: B*

A voice-message alarm can be programmed by a caregiver to alert a client when it is time to take a medication and which medications should be taken.

Incorrect Answers:

A, C, D. Use of these devices does not cue the client to take the medication at a specific time.

Reference: Padilla, R. L., Byers-Connon, S., Lohman, H. (2012). *Occupational Therapy with Elders: Strategies for the COTA*. (3rd ed.). St. Louis, MO: Elsevier Mosby. Pages 177-178.

67. *Correct Answer: C*

Clients who have paraplegia must learn compensatory strategies for cooking when seated in a wheelchair. If the client's home is equipped with a standard height stove, the placing of an angled mirror over the stove enables the client to monitor food during stove top cooking.

Incorrect Answers:

A, D. These options are not effective uses of this device.

B. This is not a safe option.

Reference: Early, M.B. (2013). *Physical Dysfunction Practice Skills for the Occupational Therapy Assistant* (3rd ed.). St. Louis, MO: Elsevier Mosby. Pages 268-269.

68. *Correct Answer: D*

Patients who have subacute rheumatoid arthritis should learn joint protection techniques. These techniques are intended to help reduce the deforming forces on the joints during daily tasks such as cooking. This knife handle allows the client to hold the knife with a stable grip and decreases the ulnar forces on the MCP joints.

Incorrect Answers:

A, C. This is not the **PRIMARY** advantage of using this type of knife.

B. A rocker knife would be indicated for one-handed cutting.

Reference: Early, M.B. (2013). *Physical Dysfunction Practice Skills for the Occupational Therapy Assistant* (3rd ed.). St. Louis, MO: Elsevier Mosby. Pages 194, 581.

69. Correct Answer: C

A patient who sustained a complete C_6 spinal cord injury typically has innervation of the radial wrist extensors. This will allow a weak tenodesis grasp. A tenodesis splint enables the patient to transfer power of active wrist extension to enable a stronger pinch. This is **MOST BENEFICIAL** for enabling the patient to hold eating utensils.

Incorrect Answers:

A. This will assist patients who have no functional use of the upper extremities.

B. A mobile arm support is used to substitute for weak proximal upper extremity strength and absent finger function.

D. A wrist cock-up splint will stabilize the wrist and interfere with the patient's ability to use a functional tenodesis grip.

Reference: Early, M.B. (2013). *Physical Dysfunction Practice Skills for the Occupational Therapy Assistant* (3rd ed.). St. Louis, MO: Elsevier Mosby. Pages 542-543, 548.

70. Correct Answer: B.

Clients who have symptoms associated with stage 2 Parkinson's disease typically have upper extremity intention tremors. The weighted fork may help the client control the movements caused by these tremors.

Incorrect Answers:

A. The primary purpose of a right-angled knife is to provide joint protection when cutting food, and would not impact the movements caused by tremors.

C. Extending the length of a utensil would increase the impact of the tremor on self-feeding.

D. The client would not be able to keep a swivel spoon steady.

Reference: Early, M.B. (2013). *Physical Dysfunction Practice Skills for the Occupational Therapy Assistant* (3rd ed.). St. Louis, MO: Elsevier Mosby. Pages 255-256.

71. Correct Answer: D

The difference in height between the toilet and the wheelchair may cause the patient to have difficulty with the transfer at the initial stages of transfer training. The COTA should assess the height of the toilet in relation to the height of the wheelchair seat. This would give the COTA information needed to make necessary environmental modifications to support the patient's ability to complete the transfer.

Incorrect Answers:

A. A bedside commode chair would not maximize the patient's independence in toileting.

B. Patient's who have an incomplete T_2 spinal cord injury are typically able to transfer independently to a variety of surfaces without assistive devices.

C. This may be completed under the direction of the OTR, but would not be the **NEXT** action the COTA should take in support of the transfer goal.

Reference: Early, M.B. (2013). *Physical Dysfunction Practice Skills for the Occupational Therapy Assistant* (3rd ed.). St. Louis, MO: Elsevier Mosby. Pages 318, 536, 550.

72. Correct Answer: A

Clients who have stage 2 Parkinson's disease typically have difficulty shifting their weight to take steps. When using a walker, the safest way for the client to turn is to stay close to the walker, stand with a wide base of support and move slowly. The client should also be taught to use a proper gait pattern to minimize fall risk.

Incorrect Answers:

B. Turning the walker and then moving the legs could cause a fall.

C. Moving the walker to one side and reaching for support could cause the client to lose balance.

D. Placing one hand on the counter and the other on the walker would provide an uneven base of support and increase the risk of falls.

Reference: Early, M.B. (2013). *Physical Dysfunction Practice Skills for the Occupational Therapy Assistant* (3rd ed.). St. Louis, MO: Elsevier Mosby. Pages 299-300, 522-524.

73. Correct Answer: B

To maintain correct hip position, the affected leg must be abducted. Placing a wedge between the legs will position the hip in neutral alignment.

Incorrect Answers:

A, C, D. These positions do not prevent adduction or rotation of the affected hip which is an essential hip precaution during this phase of recovery.

Reference: Early, M.B. (2013). *Physical Dysfunction Practice Skills for the Occupational Therapy Assistant* (3rd ed.). St. Louis, MO: Elsevier Mosby. Page 624, 630.

74. Correct Answer: C

A bed positioning program for a client who has hemiplegia should include a schedule of alternating between supine, side-lying on the affected side and side-lying on the unaffected side. The **PRIMARY** purpose of the position shown in the picture above is to promote proper alignment while side-lying on the affected side.

Incorrect Answers:

A. Although this position allows the client to move the unaffected arm, it is not the **PRIMARY** purpose for selecting this position.

B. There is no evidence indicating this position will prevent a flexor synergy.

D. The program must include a schedule of alternating positions to be effective for minimizing decubitis ulcer formation.

Reference: Early, M.B. (2013). *Physical Dysfunction Practice Skills for the Occupational Therapy Assistant* (3rd ed.). St. Louis, MO: Elsevier Mosby. Page 472.

75. Correct Answer: C

The social aspects of dining are enhanced if the residents who have hearing impairments are seated at a round table. This allows the residents to clearly see and make eye contact with others when talking.

Incorrect Answers:

A, B, D. These options are not conducive to the groups' socialization.

Reference: Padilla, R. L., Byers-Connon, S., Lohman, H. (2012). *Occupational Therapy with Elders: Strategies for the COTA.* (3rd ed.). St. Louis, MO: Elsevier Mosby. Pages 234-235.

76. Correct Answer: A

Carrying one small basket of clothes at a time reduces stress on the muscles of the back.

Incorrect Answers:

B. Large bundles of wet clothes puts unnecessary stress on the back.

C, D. Forward bending and twisting are contraindicated.

Reference: Early, M.B. (2013). *Physical Dysfunction Practice Skills for the Occupational Therapy Assistant* (3rd ed.). St. Louis, MO: Elsevier Mosby. Pages 191-193.

77. Correct Answer: B

Memory deficits and impulsivity may compromise the patient's safety during bathing tasks. A caregiver should provide stand-by assistance in order to reduce safety risk.

Incorrect Answers:

A. This patient should not stand while showering.

C. This equipment and the level of assistance is not appropriate for this patient.

D. This option does not provide enough supervision to promote the patient's safety during showering.

Reference: Early, M.B. (2013). *Physical Dysfunction Practice Skills for the Occupational Therapy Assistant* (3rd ed.). St. Louis, MO: Elsevier Mosby. Page 503.

8. Correct Answer: B

Retrograde massage techniques are effective edema management methods that can be used frequently throughout the day as part of the overall home program.

Incorrect Answers:

A. Splinting the hand at all times is contraindicated.

C. Paraffin is primarily used to decrease stiffness and relieve pain. Additionally, use of a home unit may present a safety hazard for this patient.

D. Manual lymphatic treatment techniques are used for edema from damage to the lymphatic system. These techniques require specialty training and typically are not included as part of a patient's home program.

Reference: Early, M.B. (2013). *Physical Dysfunction Practice Skills for the Occupational Therapy Assistant* (3rd ed.). St. Louis, MO: Elsevier Mosby. Page 600.

9. Correct Answer: B

The **PRIMARY** focus of the initial intervention should be for the client to learn basic personal life management skills for independent living skills and self-reliance.

Incorrect Answers:

A. Residing in a group living environment fosters dependency.

C. Engaging the client in leisure activities with friends may not support a sober/substance-free lifestyle.

D. Identifying work-related stressors does not address the client's own coping and lifestyle management strategies.

Reference: Early, M. B. (2009). *Mental Health Concepts and Techniques for the Occupational Therapy Assistant*. (4th ed.). Baltimore, MD: Wolters Kluwer – Lippincott Williams & Wilkins. Pages 160-162, 529.

30. Correct Answer: B

The **INITIAL** focus of the group should be on activities that have a high opportunity for success.

Incorrect Answers:

A. Completing a simple project may not have inherent value for the patients.

C. Interaction with others should not be the **INITIAL** focus of a group activity, but may be appropriate during the later phase of the intervention process.

D. Using OT as a diversion is an inappropriate use of services.

Reference: Early, M. B. (2009). *Mental Health Concepts and Techniques for the Occupational Therapy Assistant*. (4th ed.). Baltimore, MD: Wolters Kluwer – Lippincott Williams & Wilkins. Pages 295-297.

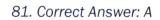

81. Correct Answer: A

Collaborating with the clients to select an activity that is valuable and meaningful would be **MOST BENEFICIAL** for supporting positive occupational performance behaviors.

Incorrect Answers:

B, C, D. These options are not client-centered and may not promote maximal participation toward the stated goal.

Reference: Early, M. B. (2009). *Mental Health Concepts and Techniques for the Occupational Therapy Assistant*. (4th ed.). Baltimore, MD: Wolters Kluwer – Lippincott Williams & Wilkins. Pages 170-171.

82. Correct Answer: B

A project group would assist the patient to feel accepted by others while engaging in valued activities that encourage cooperation and socialization.

Incorrect Answers:

A. The client has already transitioned from being self-isolative. The **MOST BENEFICIAL** group for the next level of socialization would be graded involvement in a project group.

C, D. The client should experience success within a project group before engaging in these types of groups which require higher levels of interaction and socialization skills.

Reference: Early, M. B. (2009). *Mental Health Concepts and Techniques for the Occupational Therapy Assistant*. (4th ed.). Baltimore, MD: Wolters Kluwer – Lippincott Williams & Wilkins. Pages 185, 347, 350.

83. Correct Answer: C

Encouraging the adolescent to complete the activity is setting appropriate limits and teaches the adolescent to deal with frustration in a social setting with peers.

Incorrect Answers:

A. Modifying the game rules does not promote social skills in a peer group.

B. Excusing the adolescent from the activity would only reinforce inappropriate behavior.

D. Switching to another activity would not help the adolescent deal with losing and would disrupt the group.

Reference: Solomon, J. W., O'Brien, J. C. (2011). *Pediatric Skills for Occupational Therapy Assistants*. (3rd ed.). St. Louis, MO: Elsevier Mosby. Pages 242-245.

34. *Correct Answer: D*

"Sun-downing", plus the disruptions surrounding a shift change, can cause someone who has Alzheimer's disease to become agitated and confused. Engaging the resident in a reminiscence activity related to something of value to the resident would help to redirect the resident away from the sources of confusion during this time of the day.

Incorrect Answers:

A. The resident may be too agitated to concentrate on this type of task.

B. This may feed into the resident's thoughts about leaving the facility.

C. This does not distract the resident from the activity and confusion related to the shift change.

Reference: Padilla, R. L., Byers-Connon, S., Lohman, H. (2012). *Occupational Therapy with Elders: Strategies for the COTA.* (3rd ed.). St. Louis, MO: Elsevier Mosby. Pages 278-282.

35. *Correct Answer: C*

Directing the light source from behind the client's shoulder will prevent the glare source from directing towards the client's eyes while reading magazines printed on glossy paper.

Incorrect Answers:

A, B. These do not address the client's preferred leisure activity of reading a favorite magazine.

D. The COTA should **INITIALLY** recommend modifying the lighting since this supports the client's current habits and routines for this leisure activity.

Reference: Padilla, R. L., Byers-Connon, S., Lohman, H. (2012). *Occupational Therapy with Elders: Strategies for the COTA.* (3rd ed.). St. Louis, MO: Elsevier Mosby. Page 222.

36. *Correct Answer: C*

If the state OT practice act permits the COTA to administer standardized tests, then the COTA should collaborate with the OTR to establish service competency before independently administering a manual muscle test to a client.

Incorrect Answers:

A, B. This can be completed after the OTR and COTA discuss the steps for establishing service competency.

D. This can be included as part of the plan the OTR and COTA set-up for establishing competency.

Reference: Early, M.B. (2013). *Physical Dysfunction Practice Skills for the Occupational Therapy Assistant* (3rd ed.). St. Louis, MO: Elsevier Mosby. Page 132.

87. Correct Answer: A

Since the COTA does not have recent experience in this practice setting, the COTA should have close supervision until service competency is established.

Incorrect Answers:

B. Service competency is not transferable from one job to another. The COTA must establish service competency in accordance with the policies and procedures of the new place of employment.

C. This may be used as a part of service competency; but is not the initial step.

D. Review of documentation does not provide adequate supervision.

Reference: Early, M.B. (2013). *Physical Dysfunction Practice Skills for the Occupational Therapy Assistant* (3rd ed.). St. Louis, MO: Elsevier Mosby. Pages 56-57.

88. Correct Answer: B

Supervision and structured learning provide an effective means for establishing service competency with splinting.

Incorrect Answers:

A. Attending an online professional development workshop may be useful as a first step but it does not ensure the COTA has achieved service competency to fabricate these splints.

C. Using a checklist of key tips for splinting may serve as a helpful reminder, but does not ensure service competency for fabricating splints.

D. Reviewing class notes and reading journal articles does not meet the requirement for establishing service competency in actually fabricating a splint.

Reference: Early, M.B. (2013). *Physical Dysfunction Practice Skills for the Occupational Therapy Assistant* (3rd ed.). St. Louis, MO: Elsevier Mosby. Pages 56-57.

Solomon, J. W., O'Brien, J. C. (2011). *Pediatric Skills for Occupational Therapy Assistants*. (3rd ed.). St. Louis, MO: Elsevier Mosby. Pages 6-7.

89. Correct Answer: A

In-service training as a preventive strategy benefits both staff and clients. Identifying risk factors and reducing hazards will decrease the likelihood of work-related injuries during patient transfers.

Incorrect Answers:

B, C, D. These are secondary reasons for offering nursing staff this type of in-service training. The **PRIMARY** goal is safety and injury prevention.

Reference: Sladyk, K., Jacobs, K., MacRae, N. (2010). *Occupational Therapy Essentials for Clinical Competence*. Thorofare, NJ: SLACK Inc. Page 282.

ANSWERS

90. Correct Answer: C

Non-skid footwear will help the patient obtain more secure footing and minimize the risk of falling.

Incorrect Answers:

A. Although the use of a transfer belt reduces risk, the COTA should have the patient use a cane consistent with the ambulation techniques the PT uses with the patient.

B. Providing additional caregiver support may result in dependence.

D. Walking with a shuffle gait promotes abnormal gait patterns and does not reduce the fall risk.

Reference: Early, M.B. (2013). *Physical Dysfunction Practice Skills for the Occupational Therapy Assistant* (3rd ed.). St. Louis, MO: Elsevier Mosby. Pages 298-299.

91. Correct Answer: A

Residents functioning at this cognitive level should be monitored at all times. All equipment and supplies must be returned to a storage area and accounted for prior to allowing the residents to leave the room.

Incorrect Answers:

B, C, D. These are procedural routines that may vary depending on the group and the facility.

Reference: Early, M. B. (2009). *Mental Health Concepts and Techniques for the Occupational Therapy Assistant*. (4th ed.). Baltimore, MD: Wolters Kluwer – Lippincott Williams & Wilkins. Page 328.

92. Correct Answer: C

To minimize infection risk, the client should use a personally-owned shaver. The client should use an electric razor to decrease risk of cuts from choreiform movements.

Incorrect Answers:

A. Having the client clean the razor increases the injury risk. Additionally, alcohol is not a universal germicide.

B. To minimize the risk of infection/cross contamination, personal hygiene items should not be shared.

D. Disposable straight-edge razors may be difficult for the client to use due to the choreiform movements.

Reference: Early, M.B. (2013). *Physical Dysfunction Practice Skills for the Occupational Therapy Assistant* (3rd ed.). St. Louis, MO: Elsevier Mosby. Pages 42-43, 45-46, 255-256.

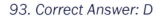

93. Correct Answer: D

Administering a developmental skills checklist after establishing service competency, is a typical responsibility for a COTA. This task is within the scope of practice for a newly certified COTA.

Incorrect Answers:

A. A sensory integration assessment requires advanced training and is typically administered and scored by an OTR.

B, C. These duties are the responsibility of an OTR.

Reference: Solomon, J. W., O'Brien, J. C. (2011). *Pediatric Skills for Occupational Therapy Assistants*. (3rd ed.). St. Louis, MO: Elsevier Mosby. Pages 6-7, 445.

94. Correct Answer: A

The COTA is obligated to provide supervision of an OT aide in accordance with specific state practice acts and governing laws.

Incorrect Answers:

B. Although it is helpful for the COTA to be familiar with specific critical demands listed on the aide's job description, the laws governing the scope of practice for OT aides supersede local policy.

C, D. These are not essential to know prior to assigning tasks to the aide.

Reference: Pendleton, H.M., Schultz-Krohn, W. (eds). (2013). *Pedretti's Occupational Therapy: Practice Skills for Physical Dysfunction* (7th ed.). St. Louis, MO: Elsevier Mosby. Page 41.

95. Correct Answer: C

To qualify for Medicare reimbursement, the documentation **MUST** indicate that the services provided are functional and medically necessary.

Incorrect Answers:

A, B, D. Documentation of these is not required to meet Medicare requirements for Reimbursement.

Reference: Padilla, R. L., Byers-Connon, S., Lohman, H. (2012). *Occupational Therapy with Elders: Strategies for the COTA*. (3rd ed.). St. Louis, MO: Elsevier Mosby. Page 72.

96. Correct Answer: A

The "A" section of the SOAP note should reflect an assessment of the situation in relation to the established goal(s). In this case the assessment is reflected **BEST** in option A.

Incorrect Answers:

B. The patient is already independent in upper extremity dressing with minimal assistance. It is unlikely the patient will require assistance for most self-care at discharge.

C. This is subjective information and should be included in the "S" section of an SOAP note.

D. This information represents an objective measure related to upper body dressing and would be best to include in the "O" section of an SOAP note.

Reference: Early, M.B. (2013). *Physical Dysfunction Practice Skills for the Occupational Therapy Assistant* (3rd ed.). St. Louis, MO: Elsevier Mosby. Pages 79-80, 90, 92.

97. Correct Answer: C

The discharge summary is a key document used when assessing outcomes. It must contain objective information about functional progress from initiation of OT to discharge.

Incorrect Answers:

A, B, D. This information is useful, but is not required in a discharge summary or when assessing outcomes.

Reference: Early, M.B. (2013). *Physical Dysfunction Practice Skills for the Occupational Therapy Assistant* (3rd ed.). St. Louis, MO: Elsevier Mosby. Pages 77, 79, 80.

98. Correct Answer: D

Emphasis of intervention in an acute mental health setting is on improving self-care skills. Progress and outcomes are based on a comparison of skills from initiation of intervention to time of discharge.

Incorrect Answers:

A. Specific job-performance skills are not addressed in an acute care facility.

B. Functional potential is typically not included in outcomes documentation.

C. Subjective impressions are not accurate indicators of outcomes.

Reference: Early, M.B. (2013). *Physical Dysfunction Practice Skills for the Occupational Therapy Assistant* (3rd ed.). St. Louis, MO: Elsevier Mosby. Pages 77, 79, 80.

Early, M. B. (2009). *Mental Health Concepts and Techniques for the Occupational Therapy Assistant.* (4th ed.). Baltimore, MD: Wolters Kluwer – Lippincott Williams & Wilkins. Pages 384, 477-478.

99. Correct Answer: B

Progress notes should provide evidence about the client's progress in relation to the established functional goals.

Incorrect Answers:

A, D. Subjective reports and progress related to other patients are not needed to justify the additional services.

C. Subjective comments about anticipated function does not provide objective evidence needed to justify additional services.

Reference: Early, M.B. (2013). *Physical Dysfunction Practice Skills for the Occupational Therapy Assistant* (3rd ed.). St. Louis, MO: Elsevier Mosby. Pages 79-80, 90.

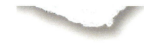

100. Correct Answer: C

Reimbursement from Medicare is determined by the number of "therapy minutes" that are documented in the minimum data set (MDS).

Incorrect Answers:

A, B, D. This information is not a requirement for reimbursement under the Medicare Prospective Payment System.

Reference: Padilla, R. L., Byers-Connon, S., Lohman, H. (2012). *Occupational Therapy with Elders: Strategies for the COTA.* (3rd ed.). St. Louis, MO: Elsevier Mosby. Pages 70-72.

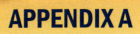
APPENDIX A:

2012 Validated Domain, Task, and Knowledge Statements for the COTA

2012 Validated Domain, Task and Knowledge Statements for the COTA

Domains are specified in bold with a two-digit number, tasks are grouped under each domain (four-digit number), and the tasks' associated knowledge statements are listed with a six-digit number.

Code	Description
01	**DOMAIN 1** **Assist the OTR to acquire information regarding factors that influence occupational performance throughout the occupational therapy process.**
0101	**Use available resources to acquire information about a client's functional skills, roles, context, and prioritized needs in order to contribute to the development of an occupational profile.**
010101	Normal development and function across the lifespan
010102	Expected patterns, progressions, and prognoses associated with conditions that limit occupational performance (e.g., stages of disease, secondary complications, outcomes)
010103	Processes and procedures for acquiring client information (e.g., client records, observation, interview, occupational profile)
010104	Types and purposes of standardized screening and assessment tools and the importance of adhering to their administration protocols
010105	Influence of client factors, context, and environments on habits, routines, roles, and rituals
010106	Methods for recognizing and responding to typical and atypical physiological, cognitive, and behavioral conditions
0102	**Provide information regarding the influence of current condition(s) and context(s) on occupational performance in order to assist the OTR in planning interventions and monitoring progress throughout the occupational therapy process.**
010201	Activity analysis in relation to the occupational profile, practice setting, and stage of occupational therapy process
010202	Internal and external influences on occupational performance (e.g., environment, context, condition, medication, other therapies)
010203	Methods for monitoring progress and recognizing indications that suggest a need for modification of the intervention plan and goals
0103	**Collaborate with the client, the client's relevant others, occupational therapy colleagues, and other professionals and staff using a client-centered approach to provide quality services guided by evidence and principles of best practice.**
010301	Influence of frames of reference and models of practice on intervention planning and activity selection
010302	Inter professional team roles, responsibilities, and care coordination (e.g., referral to and consultation with other services)
010303	Collaborative client-centered intervention and transition planning based on client skills, abilities, and expected outcomes in relation to level of service delivery and frequency and duration of intervention and available resources (includes communication with family, caregiver, and relevant others)

Code	Description
010304	Methods for advocating client and community needs (e.g., aging in place, falls prevention, health and wellness programs, community support groups, health fairs, in services)

DOMAIN 2

02	**Implement interventions in accordance with the intervention plan and under the supervision of the OTR to support client participation in areas of occupation throughout the occupational therapy process.**
0201	**Implement interventions for the infant, child, or adolescent client using clinical reasoning, the intervention plan, and best practice standards consistent with pediatric condition(s) and typical developmental milestones (e.g., motor, sensory, psychosocial, and cognitive) in order to support participation within areas of occupation.**
020101	Influence of pediatric condition(s) and typical developmental milestones on activity selection and areas of occupation
020102	Intervention activities for supporting participation in occupations based on current sensory, cognitive, motor, and psychosocial skills and abilities
020103	Strategies and procedures for facilitating or inhibiting sensory, motor, or perceptual processing based on pediatric condition(s), tasks, and environmental demands
020104	Intervention methods for improving range of motion, strength, and activity tolerance based on pediatric condition(s) in order to promote occupational performance
020105	Methods and techniques for facilitating group interventions appropriate to pediatric condition(s) and developmental level
020106	Splint fabrication and types, functions, and use of orthotic and prosthetic devices based on pediatric condition(s) and task demands
020107	Types, function, and use of assistive technology, adaptive devices, and durable medical equipment based on pediatric condition(s), task, and environmental demands
020108	Methods for adapting intervention techniques and environment based on behavioral responses and developmental needs
020109	Indications, contraindications, and technical skills for enabling feeding and eating skills based on pediatric condition(s) and developmental level
020110	Transfer and positioning techniques based on pediatric condition(s), task, and environmental demands
020111	Vocational readiness and exploration processes and procedures that support transition planning
020112	Types, functions, and use of seating options, positioning devices, and mobility systems based on pediatric condition(s), developmental level, and environmental demands
020113	Environmental modifications for maximizing accessibility and mobility in a variety of settings based on pediatric condition(s), developmental level, and task demands
020114	Methods for adapting and/or grading tasks and activities based on pediatric condition(s), developmental needs, and task demands
020115	Methods and techniques for promoting carry-over of the intervention within context based on current pediatric condition(s), developmental level, and expected outcomes (e.g., home program, caregiver instructions, teacher consultation)

Code	Description
0202	**Implement interventions for the young, middle-aged, or older adult client, using clinical reasoning, the intervention plan, and best practice standards consistent with general medical, neurological, and musculoskeletal condition(s) in order to achieve functional outcomes within areas of occupation.**
020201	Influence of general medical, neurological, and musculoskeletal condition(s) on activity selection and areas of occupation
020202	Rehabilitative strategies and procedures specific to medical, neurological, and musculoskeletal condition(s) (e.g., activities of daily living, joint protection, work simplification, energy conservation)
020203	Strategies and procedures for improving range of motion, strength, and activity tolerance based on general medical, neurological, and musculoskeletal condition(s) in order to promote occupational performance
020204	Strategies and procedures for facilitating or inhibiting sensory, motor, and perceptual processing based on general medical, neurological, and musculoskeletal condition(s)
020205	Indications, contraindications, and technical skills for effective application of superficial and deep thermal, mechanical, and electrotherapeutic physical agent modalities as an adjunct to participation in an activity
020206	Splint fabrication and types, functions, and use of orthotic and prosthetic devices based on client needs; general medical, neurological, and musculoskeletal condition(s); and task demands
020207	Types, functions, and use of assistive technology (i.e., high and low tech), adaptive devices, and durable medical equipment based on client needs and general medical, neurological, and musculoskeletal condition(s)
020208	Indications, contraindications, and technical skills for enabling feeding and eating based on client needs and general medical, neurological, and musculoskeletal condition(s)
020209	Transfer methods and positioning techniques based on client needs; general medical, neurological, and musculoskeletal condition(s); task; and environmental demands
020210	Types, functions, and use of seating options, positioning devices, and mobility systems based on client needs; general medical, neurological, and musculoskeletal condition(s); task; and environmental demands
020211	Environmental modifications for maximizing accessibility and mobility in a variety of settings based on client needs; general medical, neurological, and musculoskeletal condition(s); and task demands
020212	Ergonomic principles and universal design for health promotion and injury prevention
020213	Methods for adapting and grading tasks and activities based on client needs and medical, neurological, and musculoskeletal condition(s)
020214	Methods and techniques for promoting carry-over of the intervention within context based on current medical condition(s) and expected outcomes (e.g., home program, caregiver instructions)
0203	**Implement interventions for the young, middle-aged, and older adult client, using clinical reasoning, the intervention plan, and best practice standards consistent with psychosocial, cognitive, and developmental abilities in order to achieve functional outcomes within areas of occupation.**
020301	Influence of psychosocial, cognitive, and developmental abilities on activity selection and areas of occupation
020302	Methods and techniques for facilitating group interventions appropriate to participants' psychosocial, cognitive, and developmental abilities
020303	Approaches (e.g., remediation, compensation, prevention) and interventions (e.g., problem solving, medication management, memory strategies) appropriate for psychosocial and cognitive models of practice (e.g., cognitive behavioral, behavioral, acquisitional, developmental)

Code	Description
020304	Environmental modifications to enhance community safety and well-being consistent with occupational roles and client needs
020305	Types, functions, and use of assistive technology and adaptive devices based on psychosocial, cognitive, and developmental abilities
020306	Methods and techniques for adapting and grading intervention activities based on psychosocial, cognitive, and developmental abilities
020307	Methods and techniques for promoting carry-over of the intervention within context based on psychosocial, cognitive, and developmental abilities (e.g., home program, caregiver instructions, job coach)

DOMAIN 3

03	**Uphold professional standards and responsibilities to promote quality in practice.**
0301	**Maintain and enhance competence by participating in professional development activities and applying learned content as relevant to job role, practice setting, and regulatory body in order to provide effective services guided by evidence.**
030101	Methods for engaging in professional development and service competency activities (e.g., peer review, supervisory meeting, self-assessment)
030102	Methods of accessing, reviewing, and applying professional literature to practice
0302	**Provide ethical and safe occupational therapy services in collaboration with the OTR and in accordance with applicable regulations, laws, facility policies and procedures, and accreditation guidelines governing practice in order to protect consumers.**
030201	Policies, procedures, and guidelines related to service delivery
030202	Licensure laws, federally mandated requirements, reimbursement policies, and accreditation guidelines related to occupational therapy service delivery (e.g., client confidentiality, levels of supervision, plan of care certification/recertification, referral policy)
030203	Safety concerns and risk management
030204	Continuous quality improvement processes and procedures
030205	Scope of practice and practice standards for occupational therapy (e.g., supervision of aides and volunteers, role delineation)
030206	Accountability processes and procedures (e.g., documentation guidelines, components of an intervention plan, coding systems, electronic medical records, written documentation)

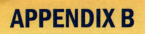

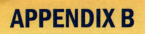

APPENDIX B:
References

ACOTE. (2011). *Accreditation Standards for an Associate-Degree-Level Educational Program for the Occupational Therapy Assistant*. American Occupational Therapy Association.

*Barnhart PA. (1997). *The Guide to National Professional Certification Programs* (2nd ed.). Amherst, MA:HRD Press.

Boyt Schell B, Gillen G, Scaffa M, Cohn E. (2014). *Willard and Spackman's Occupational Therapy* (12th ed.). Philadelphia, PA: Lippincott Williams & Wilkins.

*Brookfield S. (1987). *Developing Critical Thinkers*. San Francisco, CA: Jossey-Bass, Inc.

Case-Smith J, O'Brien J. (2010). *Occupational Therapy for Children* (6th ed.). St. Louis, MO: Elsevier Mosby

Coppard BM & Lohman H. (2008). *Introduction to Splinting: A Clinical-Reasoning & Problem Solving Approach* (3rd ed.). St. Louis, MO: Elsevier Mosby.

*Covey SR. (1989). *The 7 Habits of Highly Effective People*. New York: Simon & Schuster.

Davis CM. (2011). *Patient Practitioner Interaction: An Experiential Manual for Developing the Art of Health Care* (5th ed.). Thorofare, NJ: SLACK, Inc.

Delany JV, Pendzick PJ. (2009). *Working with Children and Adolescents: A Guide for the Occupational Therapy Assistant*. Upper Saddle River, NJ: Pearson-Prentice Hall.

Early MB. (2009). *Mental Health Concepts and Techniques for the Occupational Therapy Assistant* (4th ed.). Baltimore, MD: Wolters Kluwer –Lippincott, Williams & Wilkins.

Early MB, (2013). *Physical Dysfunction: Practice Skills for the Occupational Therapy Assistant* (3rd ed.). St Louis, MO: Elsevier Mosby.

Keough J, Sain S, Roller C. (2011). *Kinesiology for the Occupational Therapy Assistant: Essential Components of Function and Movement*. Thorofare, NJ: SLACK Inc.

*McClain N, Richardson B, & Wyatt J. (2004, May-June). *A profile of certification for pediatric nurses. Pediatric Nursing*, 207-211.

Meriano C & Latella D. (2008). *Occupational Therapy Interventions, Function and Occupations*. Thorofare, NJ: Slack, Inc.

*Microsoft (2003). *Microsoft certifications benefits of certification*. Retrieved from www.microsoft.com/traincert.

NBCOT, Inc. (2013). *2013 Certification Renewal Handbook*. Gaithersburg, MD: NBCOT 2013 Publications.

Padilla RL, Byers-Connon S, Lohman H. (eds). (2012) *Occupational Therapy with Elders: Strategies for the COTA* (3rd ed.). St. Louis, MO: Elsevier Mosby.

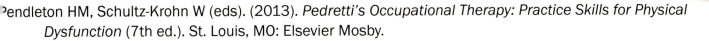

Pendleton HM, Schultz-Krohn W (eds). (2013). *Pedretti's Occupational Therapy: Practice Skills for Physical Dysfunction* (7th ed.). St. Louis, MO: Elsevier Mosby.

Radomski MV, Trombly-Latham C. (2008). *Occupational Therapy for Physical Dysfunction* (6th ed.). Baltimore, MD: Lippincott, Williams and Wilkins.

Sladyk K, Jacobs K, MacRae N. (2010). *Occupational Therapy Essentials for Clinical Competence.* Thorofare, NJ: SLACK Inc.

Smith-Gabai H. (2011). *Occupational Therapy in Acute Care.* Bethesda, MD: AOTA Press.

Solomon J, O'Brien J. (2011). *Pediatric Skills for Occupational Therapy Assistants* (3rd ed.). St. Louis, MO: Elsevier Mosby.

Taylor R. (2008). *The Intentional Relationship: Occupational Therapy and Use of Self.* Philadelphia, PA: FA Davis.

Wagenfeld A, Kaldenberg J. (2005). *Foundations of Pediatric Practice for the Occupational Therapy Assistant.* Thorofare, NJ: SLACK Inc.

* References cited during introductory chapter of this study guide. These references should not be viewed as examination item references.

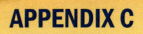

APPENDIX C:
Abbreviations and Acronyms

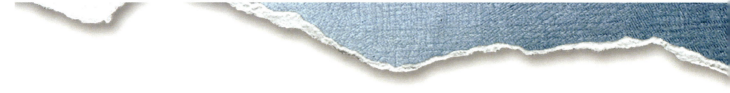

The following is a list of abbreviations and acronyms that may be used in examination items. Please note: The list provided in this Appendix is intended for study purposes only and is not comprehensive.

Abbreviation or Acronym	Expansion
ADA	The Americans with Disabilities Act
ADL	Activities of daily living
AIDS	Acquired immunodeficiency syndrome
ALS	Amyotrophic lateral sclerosis
BADL	Basic activities of daily living
COPD	Chronic obstructive pulmonary disease
COTA	CERTIFIED OCCUPATIONAL THERAPY ASSISTANT COTA®
CPR	Cardiopulmonary resuscitation
CRPS	Complex regional pain syndrome
CVA	Cerebrovascular accident
DIP	Distal interphalangeal*
DSM 5	Diagnostic and Statistical Manual of Mental Disorders – 5th Edition
HIPAA	Health Insurance Portability and Accountability Act
HIV	Human immunodeficiency virus
IADL	Instrumental activities of daily living
IDEA	Individuals with Disabilities Education Act
IEP	Individualized Education Program
MCP	Metacarpophalangeal*
OTR	OCCUPATIONAL THERAPIST REGISTERED OTR®
PIP	Proximal interphalangeal*
ROM	Range of motion
SCI	Spinal cord injury
SOAP	Subjective, Objective, Assessment, Plan (components of the problem-oriented medical record)

*Must be followed by the word "joint"

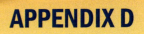
APPENDIX D:

Listing of common:

Diagnoses/Conditions

Intervention Applications/Equipment

Service Delivery Components

Roles and Responsibilities

Practice Settings

The following is a list of diagnoses/condition, intervention applications/equipment, service delivery components and setting that may be used as part of a multiple-choice examination item or clinical simulation problem. Please note: The lists provided in this Appendix are intended for study purposes only and are not comprehensive.

Diagnoses/Conditions

- Attention deficit hyperactivity disorder (ADHD)
- Acquired immunodeficiency syndrome (AIDS)
- Adjustment disorders
- Alcohol/substance abuse
- Alzheimer's disease
- Amyotrophic lateral sclerosis (ALS)
- Amputations (upper and lower extremity)
- Anxiety disorders
- Aphasia
- Apraxia (ideomotor/ideational)
- Arthritis (osteoarthritis/rheumatoid arthritis)
- Ataxia
- Autonomic dysreflexia
- Back pain
- Bipolar disorder
- Burns
- Cardiac/Cardiopulmonary disease
- Cerebral palsy
- Cerebrovascular Accident (CVA)
- Chronic Obstructive Pulmonary Disease (COPD)
- Cognitive dysfunction
- Complex regional pain syndrome (CRPS)
- Cumulative trauma disorders
  - deQuervain's tenosynovitis
  - Carpal tunnel syndrome
  - Lateral epicondylitis
  - Cubital tunnel syndrome
- Death and dying
- Decubitis ulcers
- Deep vein thrombosis
- Dementia/Alzheimer's disease/memory loss
- Depression
- Development (normal/abnormal)
- Developmental disorders
  - Autism spectrum disorder
  - Developmental delay
  - Down syndrome
- Diabetes
- Domestic violence/Abuse (child/spousal/elder)
- Dysphagia
- Dyspraxia
- Eating disorders
  - Anorexia
  - Bulimia
  - Obesity
- Edema
- Encephalopathy
- Failure to thrive
- Fall risk

- Fetal alcohol syndrome
- Fibromyalgia
- Fractures (upper and lower extremity)
- Guillain-Barré syndrome
- Hand injury
- Hemiplegia/hemiparesis
- Heterotropic ossification
- Human Immunodeficiency Virus (HIV)
- Hypertension/hypotension
- Hypertonia/spasticity
- Hypotonicity/flaccidity
- Intellectual disability
- Ischemia
- Joint replacement (hip/knee)
- Joints (MCP /PIP/DIP)
- Learning disabilities
- Low vision
- Muscular dystrophy
- Medication management (side effects)
- Multiple sclerosis
- Myasthenia gravis
- Nerve injuries/peripheral neuropathy
  - Median
  - Radial
  - Ulnar
- Normal child development
- Obsessive compulsive disorder (OCD)
- Oral motor dysfunction
- Osteoporosis
- Pain management
- Paralysis
- Parkinson's disease
- Perceptual disorders
- Perseveration
- Personality disorders
- Post-polio syndrome
- Post traumatic stress disorder (PTSD)
- Postural hypotension
- Reading disorders
- Respiratory disorders
- Schizophrenia
- Spinal cord injuries (levels of injury)
  - Paraplegia
  - Tetraplegia
  - Quadriplegia
- Scar remodeling
  - Hypertrophic scar
  - Wound healing
- Sensory modulation deficits
- Spasticity

- Spina bifida
- Substance use/abuse
- Suicidal ideation
- Tactile defensiveness
- Tardive dyskinesia
- Tendon injury/repair (hand)
- Traumatic brain injury (TBI)
- Tonic bite
- Vision impairments
  - Homonymous hemianopsia
  - Low vision
  - Macular degeneration
  - Retinopathy
  - Visual field deficits
- Work-related injuries
- Wound healing (stages)

ntervention Applications/Equipment

- Activities of daily living (ADL)
- Adaptive equipment
- Aging in place
- Allen Cognitive Levels
- Assessment tools (standardized and non-standardized)
- Assistive devices
- Assistive technology (low tech/high tech)
- Augmentative and alternative communication
- Balance training/retraining
- Behavior management strategies
- Biomechanical model
- Body mechanics
- Body scheme awareness
- Cardiac rehabilitation (activities/phases)
- Chaining
  - Forward chaining
  - Backward chaining
- Client-centered approaches
- Cognitive–perceptual intervention strategies
- Community integration
- Community mobility
- Community referrals
- Compensatory techniques
- Coping strategies
- Desensitization techniques
- Developmental play
- Discharge planning
- Durable medical equipment
- Edema management
- Energy conservation
- Endurance exercises
- Environmental adaptation/modification
- Environmental control units (uses/indications)
- Ergonomic principles
- Errorless learning
- Evidence-based practice
- Feeding/swallowing
- Flexibility/stretching exercises

- Functional ambulation
- Goal-setting and prioritization (in collaboration with OTR)
- Graded activities
- Grasp development/grasp patterns
- Group dynamics/group facilitation
- Handwriting/pre-writing skills
- Home program education
- Injury prevention (educational programming)
- Information gathering strategies
- Interprofessional team collaboration
- Joint protection techniques
- Just-right challenge
- Lifestyle modification
- Memory strategies
- Mobility training
- Motor skills/motor control/motor planning
- Muscle testing
- Observation techniques
- Occupational profile development
- Oral motor skills
- Pain management techniques
- Patient/caregiver education
- Perceptual skill development
- Physical agent modalities (indications/contraindications)
- Positioning (techniques and devices)
- Pressure garments
- Prosthetics (types/functions/uses)
- Purposeful activity
- Range of motion (testing/exercises)
- Reflexes
  - Asymmetrical tonic neck reflex (ATNR)
  - Symmetrical tonic neck reflex (STNR)
  - Labyrinthine
  - Head righting
- Relaxation training
- Risk management (related to service delivery)
- Role playing
- Safety precautions (client and caregiver)
- Seating (types and devices)
- Sensory modulation techniques
- Sensory testing
- Sensory reeducation
- Service competency
- Sequencing skills and abilities
- Social skills
- Splint/orthotic (fabrication/modification)
- Strengthening exercises
- Stress management
- Transfer training/education
- Transition planning
- Trunk control
- Universal design
- Universal precautions
- Visual motor skill development
- Vocational training

- Wellness educational programming
- Wheelchair assessment/modification
- Wheelchair (functional mobility)
- Work hardening/functional capacity
- Work simplification
- Workplace modification

Service Delivery Components (Occupational Therapy Process)

- Activity analysis
- Activity selection
- Assessment in collaboration with OTR (standardized/non standardized)
- Clinical observation
- Communication skills
- Components of an intervention plan
- Confidentiality
- Conflict of interest
- Conflict resolution

Roles and Responsibilities

- Cultural sensitivity/diversity
- Culturally responsive care
- COTA/OTR roles and responsibilities
- Continuous quality improvement/performance improvement planning
- Discharge planning (processes and procedures)
- Documentation
- Evidence-based practice
- Federally mandated requirements for service delivery
- Frames of reference/models of practice
- Goal-setting/prioritization (in collaboration with OTR)
- Informed consent
- Insurance authorization/reimbursement
- Intervention planning
- Interviewing skills/methods
- Interprofessional team process
- Listening
- Negotiating
- Outcomes measures
- Professional development activities
- Professional liability
- Program evaluation
- Promoting the profession
- Research methods
- Interpretation of results (in collaboration with OTR)
- Resource management
  - Time
  - Equipment
  - Supplies
- Risk management
- Screening (standardized/non standardized)
- Service collaboration
- Service competencies

- Scope of practice
- Strategic planning/goals
- Supervision

Settings/Situations

- Acute care hospital
- Adult day-care center
- ADA
- Architectural/environmental barriers
- Assisted living facilities
- Automobile
- Bathing/bathroom mobility
- Classroom
- Clinic
- Cooking/meal preparation
- Community-based settings
- Consultant
- Day-care facility
- Dressing
- Early childhood intervention
- Eating/dining
- Grooming/hygiene
- Groups (inpatient/outpatient)
- Group home
- Home health
- Hospice
- IDEA
- Independence
- Inpatient rehabilitation facility
- Interests
- Job site/vocational/prevocational
- Leisure activities
- Long term care facility
- Playground
- Play activities
- Preschool
- Prison/confinement facility
- School-based
- Skilled nursing facility
- Volunteers
- Wellness programs
- Workplace